AFTA SpringerBriefs in Family Therapy

Series Editor

Carmen Knudson-Martin
Education & Counseling, Rogers Hall
Lewis & Clark Grad School
Portland, OR, USA

SpringerBriefs present concise summaries of cutting-edge research and practical applications. Featuring compact volumes of 50 to 125 pages, the series covers a range of content from professional to academic. Typical topics might include: A timely report of state-of-the art analytical techniques A bridge between new research results, as published in journal articles, and a contextual literature review A snapshot of a hot or emerging topic An in-depth case study or clinical example A presentation of core concepts that students must understand in order to make independent contributions

Gita Seshadri • Dumayi Gutierrez

Interracial, Intercultural, and Interfaith Couples and Families Across the Life Cycle

A Clinician's Guide

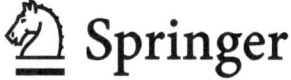 Springer

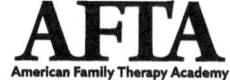

Gita Seshadri ⓘ
Alliant International University
Sacramento, CA, USA

Dumayi Gutierrez ⓘ
Alliant International University
San Diego, CA, USA

ISSN 2196-5528   ISSN 2196-5536   (electronic)
AFTA SpringerBriefs in Family Therapy
ISBN 978-3-031-58537-1   ISBN 978-3-031-58538-8   (eBook)
https://doi.org/10.1007/978-3-031-58538-8

This Springer imprint is published by the registered company Springer Nature Switzerland AG
The registered company address is: Gewerbestrasse 11, 6330 Cham, Switzerland

If disposing of this product, please recycle the paper.

We dedicate this book to all combinations of Interracial, Intercultural, Interfaith Families. We See You

Series Foreword

The AFTA Springer Briefs in Family Therapy is an official publication of the American Family Therapy Academy. Each volume focuses on the practice and policy implications of innovative systemic research and theory in family therapy and allied fields. Our goal is to make information about families and systemic practices in societal contexts widely accessible in a reader friendly, conversational, and practical style. AFTA's core commitment to equality, social responsibility, and justice are represented in each volume.

In this volume, Gita Seshadri and Dumayi Gutierrez explore the multiple contextual levels interracial and intercultural couples navigate as they negotiate the various developmental stages of their life cycle. Using Bronfenbrenner's ecological model as a contextual framework and a social constructionist approach to what it means to create an interracial/intercultural relationship, Seshadri and Gutierrez expand beyond the problem-focused, primarily White-Black heterosexual way this topic has usually been addressed to offer an inclusive, comprehensive, strength-based lens that addresses intersections of race, culture, sexuality, gender, and religion and offers useful clinical interventions.

Recognizing that acceptance of "mixed" relationships is increasing at the same time as race itself is politically charged and divisions in societies appear to be solidifying, the authors tackle how interracial/intercultural couples respond to societal issues such as discrimination and marginalization and address privilege, fairness, and equity within their own relationships. Chapters enable readers to consider the developmental tasks and opportunities afforded to interracial/intercultural couples from attraction to retirement, with illustrative case examples reflective of their diversity.

Carmen Knudson-Martin, Series Editor
AFTA Springer Briefs in Family Therapy
Portland, Oregon, USA

AFTA Springer Briefs in Family Therapy

A Publication of the American Family Therapy Academy

Founded in 1977, the American Family Therapy Academy is a non-profit organization of leading family therapy teachers, clinicians, program directors, policymakers, researchers, and social scientists dedicated to advancing systemic thinking and practices for families in their social context.

Vision

AFTA envisions a just world by transforming social contexts that promote health, safety, and well-being of all families and communities.

Mission

AFTA's mission is developing, researching, teaching, and disseminating progressive, just family therapy and family-centered practices and policies.

Acknowledgments

Interracial, Intercultural, and Interfaith Couples and Families Across the Life Cycle: A Clinician's Guide is a guide for clinicians and educators. We utilize Bronfenbrenner's Ecological Systems model and various framework to highlight various experiences and sociocultural influences that these relationships face throughout their lifetime. As authors, we highlight historical and recent research regarding these relationships and provide various clinical examples throughout.

We are truly grateful for the mentorship of Carmen Knudson-Martin, the Series Editor of AFTA Spring Briefs in Family Therapy, and the opportunity to come together to create this book. Through her advice, constructive feedback, and warmth, we developed a strong foundation to this book and grew exponentially as authors alongside it.

We want to give an in-depth thank you to our families who supported us through this journey. As two Women of Color, both strengthening and building our foundation of our careers, the unwavering patience and flexibility of our loved ones have helped us through each chapter, challenge, and triumph we faced.

Gita: To my significant other, you helped me in more ways than you know. Intellectual conversations, discussions of personal experiences, helpful and frustrating debates, growth, empathy, and kindness, and hours in front of the computer. Thank you for your willingness to create space and support me through this venture. To my parents/family, thank you for letting me focus on this and take hours/days/ months away from you to support this project. To my co-author Dumayi, thank you for our collegial relationship, mentorship, and friendship. I so appreciate you, your patience, time/energy, and your perspective of this work! You helped to develop this into something that we are both proud of! Thank you so much!

Dumayi: To my wife, you're my rock and I wouldn't be an accomplished scholar, professor, therapist, and mother without you. To my daughters, everyday my work is dedicated to you, to contribute to building a world of justice, equity, and inclusion so you may thrive as you desire. To my parents, siblings, and abuela, thank you for your love. Without our bond, I wouldn't be the professional I am today. Lastly, to my fantastic co-author Gita, I thank you for asking me to be part of this journey. I have grown immensely in this process, am in awe of your work, and am happy to say we did it!!

Our special thanks also goes out to one of our first literacy editors, Deborah Dallinger, who provided guidance on refinement and clarity as book writers. Lastly, thank you to the American Family Therapy Academy and the Springer publication team for the opportunity to contribute to social justice through our work with intercultural, interracial, and interfaith partners and relationships.

Contents

About the Editors

Gita Seshadri is an Associate Professor in the Couple and Family Therapy Program at Alliant International University in Sacramento and Online campuses. As of 2022, she assumed the role of Branch Director at the Sacramento campus. She has a passion for working with multiple diverse communities. She has published and presented nationally and internationally on interracial and intercultural couples and families, on various topics of diversity (South Asian topics/Women of Color), intersectionality, process-based qualitative research, mentoring, and emotion management. Much of her clinical work and experience encompasses intercultural, interracial, partners and families, parent-child relationships, couples, and sexually diverse populations.

Dumayi Gutierrez is an Assistant Professor in the Couple and Family Therapy Program at Alliant International University in San Diego and Online campuses. She has a passion for working with multiple diverse communities. She has published and presented nationally on minority stress, intersectionality of self and family systems, couple support systems, resiliencies of sexually diverse and gender expansive Latine/x populations, intersectional and cultural humble care, and Women of Color in higher education. She uses a narrative, experiential, and feminist approach, utilizing techniques of advocacy and empowerment. Much of her clinical work and experience encompasses intercultural, interracial, sexually, and gender diverse partners and families.

Chapter 1
Introduction to an Interracial Relationship: Where Do We Situate Ourselves?

> *"Cultural patterns of oppression are not only interrelated but are bound together and influenced by the intersectional systems of society. Examples of this include race, gender, class, ability, and ethnicity" Kimberlé Williams Crenshaw*
>
> Collins (2000, p. 42)

The topic of interracial and intercultural marriages and relationships has been a topic of interest throughout the centuries. The number of new marriages that were interracial (i.e., differing race) increased by 16% from 1967 to 2019, whereas intraracial (i.e., same race) marriages decreased by that same percentage. Public approval for interracial marriages has also increased by 89% since the 1950s (Livingston, 2017; MCarthy, 2021; Parker & Barroso, 2021). When exploring attitudes toward interracial marriage, the divorce rate, discrimination, and other topics related to the interracial experience, previous research has focused primarily on relationships among those of Black or African American descent and those of White backgrounds. However, more and more people of differing backgrounds are choosing to intermarry, and face interracially specific issues based on their particular intercultural and interracial mixing; for example, Black-Hispanic relationships have a higher risk of dissolution (Brown et al., 2018). There are also those who have preference for choosing White partners over POC, people of color (e.g., Asian or Black), to interracially date because of various biases (Buggs, 2019). According to the US Census Bureau (2018), interracial marriages among seven different racial combinations have increased by 2.8% between the years 2000 and 2012–2016.

With the influx of various cultures across the United States and worldwide, questions around relationship and couplehood abound, as the intraracial (i.e., same race) models of relationships don't work for interracial and intercultural couples. The assumption about these relationships is that there is primarily one way of doing things, the way that everyone does, like an objective truth to how relationships work. In reality, this creates more consternation and shows a lack of creativity while ignoring the influence of race, culture, and religion, without being collaborative or inclusive. Interracial, intercultural, and interfaith relationships bring questions about how couples and families negotiate aspects of culture, diversity, and

© American Family Therapy Academy (AFTA) 2024
G. Seshadri, D. Gutierrez, *Interracial, Intercultural, and Interfaith Couples and Families Across the Life Cycle*, AFTA SpringerBriefs in Family Therapy, https://doi.org/10.1007/978-3-031-58538-8_1

difference across various developmental stages in their life cycle. Specifically, how do couples manage differing cultures, and even differing faiths in a relationship among racial differences, and how do they manage this across the life cycle?

What's the Problem?

Although attitudes are changing, there still appears to be a primarily negative attitude toward interracial and intercultural couple relationships. There is frequently a lack of acceptance from society and family members that is often substantially rooted in racism and prejudice. There may also be a genuine belief that individuals from different backgrounds cannot authentically fall in love and create a strong relationship due to cultural and racial differences. A belief by some that there is a hidden agenda behind choosing to be in an interracial marriage, rather than true love for each other, may also stigmatize interracial relationships as negative experiences (e.g., marrying for status or money, rather than love) or not having satisfying marriages.

Lastly, in our world today and the ever-changing political landscape, race has become a politically charged issue. Policy issues related to immigration or racial advocacy movements have reinforced the tension around interracial couples and families infinitely, where now both partners in a relationship can be further ostracized (Schueths, 2014). In addition, more and more in our society are asking us to explore diversity, equity, and inclusion within our workplaces and relationships. With this, people are asking more of their coworkers, organizations, relationships, spouses, and children to acknowledge equity, disparity, privilege, and oppression.

Even potentially unrelated topics, like the overturning of Roe vs Wade by the Supreme Court, have introduced fears around how it will impact interracial marriage (Ciesemier & Goodwin, 2022). While this may appear an unrelated issue, this topic can be deeply interwoven within the life cycle as it relates to children, dating, and marriage and can show up in both direct and indirect ways, such as stereotypes and/or microaggressions.

Although some feel additional openness to engage in interracial relationships, positive attitudes and acceptance toward interracial relationships are limited by stereotypes and social messages (Bratter & Eschbach, 2006; Hibbler & Shinew, 2002; Lewandowski & Jackson, 2001; Mills & Daly, 1995; Solsberry, 1994). Media-perpetuated myths, varying acceptance in different racial groups, and a higher divorce rate all contribute to a negative attitude regarding the subject (Bratter & King, 2008; Fu et al., 2001; Killian, 2003; Solsberry, 1994). In the past, discrimination toward those in interracial relationships was more visible; whereas now, the manifestation of prejudice may be hidden and covert (Mills & Daly, 1995; Nemoto, 2004). Covert prejudice or concealed forms of discrimination still occur. For example, a couple must decide visibility or invisibility or affection vs. pretending to be friends only, believing that the public sphere is unsafe, which is mediated by public places or other discourses (Steinbugler, 2005; Sullivan, 2005; Thompson & Collier, 2006). The strategy employed to survive is often codeswitching, which is implementing behavior to assimilate to the situation and blend in. While attempting to survive in these moments, the couple doesn't get to move beyond this phase of questioning how they are *surviving*. This inevitably becomes problematic between the partners in the relationship and with others.

What Do We Do with the "Social Instructions" of Life Stages?

Although same-race and interracial couples face the same life transitions as other couples, such as (in no particular order) attraction, dating, cohabitation, marriage, parenting/children, launching, and retirement, for interracial couples, these transitions are especially pivotal in identity and relationship development. These transitions are often potential areas of conflict due to navigating differing and sometimes opposing cultural traditions; political, sexual, and religious nuances also play a role. For example, in the paragraph above, how might a couple navigate the public sphere after having children? Would the strategy change from when the couple was married and before children? How would they distinguish between codeswitching for survival vs. being themselves?

Social instructions, which carry "shoulds" and prescribed ways of being abound, and can bring a couple together or become sources of tension; couples can struggle around relationship strategies and with their relationship structure (Seshadri & Knudson-Martin, 2013). Not surprisingly, this all leads to the perception and feeling that there is a great level of instability and social isolation plaguing interracial relationships, leaving mental health professionals helpless as to what to do to help their interracial and intercultural clients, even when the issues are not directly related to culture. In addition, how will they help the couple interact with other systems of relationship (i.e., family members, neighbors, community, and society)? What do we need to consider?

Race

When considering race, many assume that this is an inherent type of categorization that doesn't include expectations or implied instructions or shoulds. From a social constructionist perspective, race is a constructed category that becomes meaningful to the people involved and to the larger society through processes of categorization and labeling of individuals based on appearance. Race is also part of a personal identity and can be personalized through culture and ethnicity. Racial identity changes through the mixing of races more often than mixing cultures, because it results in a varied biological appearance from a combination of multiple backgrounds. A hierarchy becomes automatic when there is a group that functions as the majority and the minorities do not have enough power to have a socially "valid" opinion.

Across the world, colorism has focused on lighter being more prized in beauty, attraction, wealth (e.g., having enough money to not be working class/being in the sun/getting tanned/darker), etc. In this sense, lighter skin tones became more privileged (Shankar & Subish, 2016). When an interracial couple walks down the street and there are visible differences in skin color and other biological features, this plays a role in power, status, and the sociocultural environment. Focusing on race as a socially constructed phenomenon allows analyses of the societal and relational processes involved as partners make meaning of and personalize race, ethnicity, and culture, rather than assuming that the idea of race is an objective reality. Should we also take the same stance with a view of culture?

Culture and Religion

Culture plays a large role in the organization of society and in people's lives; it describes the meaning that people attribute to the realities they have had in their lives around culture (Paré, 1996). Specifically, a culture is "a group of persons who share particular interpretations of the world because of reasons of geography, gender, religion, and other contingencies that play a role in lending a degree of homogeneity to their perspectives" (Paré, 1996, p. 25). This is vital to understanding interracial couples' experiences because it explains previous histories that the couple brings to the relationship and explores previous traditions and ways of growing up. For example, a well-known holiday in the United States is Christmas, with origins in the Christian faith; what shoulds are there for a White South Asian interracial, intercultural, and interreligious couple during the December holiday season? White culture and Christianity suggest that gifts, Santa (for children), and Christmas trees are put up and celebrated, and maybe going to church; South Asian Hindu culture would not recognize this holiday, because this is not in their religious tradition. With or without religion, what would the shoulds or instructions be during the December holiday season? What would this look like? How might they interact with others around these traditions?

Intermixing Interracial, Intercultural, and Interfaith Differences

Although related in definition, race, ethnicity, culture, and religion capture different aspects of the human experience. It is important to make a distinction; in this book, interracial couples will most likely include both interracial and intercultural differences, and sometimes even interfaith differences. It is important to highlight experiences of interracial couples who look similar despite cultural differences (i.e., White couple–one Irish, one Greek) will likely have different experiences than those who do not (an Asian-African American couple–one Chinese, one African American). It is also important to note that while White-African American couples were and are the most researched of all mixed couplings and are said to be the most taboo of all interracial combinations (Childs, 2004), we will be using their background and backdrop of research for this book, while creating a foundation for other mixed couplings around race and culture. This book will center on the diversity of interracial, intercultural, and interfaith dynamics. It is our hope that the reader will continue to think about how the racial, cultural, and religious nuances of the partners sitting in front of them are nuanced not only in experiences but also in physical makeup.

Conceptualizing Systemic Influences

While the trend is moving toward more acceptance and understanding of interracial/intercultural marriages in general, there are still experiences of covert discrimination, which suggests that prejudice and discrimination remain significant to the experiences of these couples. Seshadri and Knudson-Martin (2013) outlined a systemic analysis regarding how discrimination may affect the couple through their relationships, friends, neighborhood, communities, and society. Recent literature also suggests that interracial relationships may be shifting toward ideals requiring more fairness (Han, 2021). However, issues of fairness can be a loaded word in considering privilege; fairness suggests that all parties come to the table equally with resources, when often this is not always the case. In effect, we choose to refer to these discussions and questions as issues of equity instead. In the past, when intermarrying with Whites, the minority partner would be expected to acculturate; now, the desire and demand is increasingly that there is equal participation in the culture of both partners, or the partner with most of the privilege acknowledge their status in the relationship and how they contribute to the relationship in terms of power, while even taking a step back. There is a demand for acknowledgment that the relational and social environments have a role in this context.

Clinical literature suggests acknowledging these hidden and covert messages more openly; therapists who work with interracial and intercultural couples need to acknowledge their own roles (therapist's bias) and beliefs to challenge those roles and beliefs by others and society (Killian, 2002). In addition, they need to explore hidden messages that the families send to each other regarding culture through assessment tools. Despite decreased negativity toward interracial/intercultural marriages, there is little guidance available to these couples. This suggests the need for more strength-based research focused on understanding their experiences, as well as a need for useful interventions for mental health professionals in the field, and understanding of how they contribute to an interracial, intercultural, and interfaith couple's dynamic. To incorporate a strength-based perspective, social constructionism and ecological systems theory function as guiding frameworks.

Social Constructionism

Social constructionism describes social understandings as constructed by the people who live in the society of interest; rather than believing that entities are inherently what they are by their description and function, these entities become what they are through language and human construction of what humans believe the object or circumstances to be, and this becomes what people believe. For example, the term "interracial" has been constructed as a relationship that includes members of different genotypic features, yet if the word "race" was not collectively defined and part of our language and reality, this term would not make sense. Thus, notions of identity, self, and emotion—all important to understanding the experience of interracial couples—are best understood as relational processes. Dialogue between partners carries the history of the relationship which manifests in every action, which helps to establish credibility, continuity, and morality within the relationship (Gergen, 2015).

From a social constructionist view, the personal experiences of each individual cannot be referred to as private experiences or reflections due to the influences of culture, language, events, and other societal processes and collective accounts (Gergen, 2015). Relationship identity is thus socially constructed. A couple's identity is fluid and shaped through relationships, meaning, and context. A couple negotiates their identity through meaning ascribed to their experiences. Coherent meanings are understandable to those within the relationship and keep a relationship together (Gergen, 2015). Further, emotions are relational rather than an individual process. They arise within a particular context and function in a relationship by performance and action, are readable to other people through patterns, and create social meaning and context to the relationship (Gergen, 2015).

Constructing Couplehood/Partnerships

Berger and Kellner (1994) emphasized that marriage is a major site of social construction processes as partners integrate their individual experiences to create a shared meaning and structure their lives. Through this pivotal relationship, ongoing validation of personhood and standing is contributed by significant others to create security in the relationship. The process of becoming a couple presents the negotiation of many aspects in a relationship: economic; emotional; spiritual and religious; power; physical power; couple/marital identity; boundaries with friends, family, in-laws, community, and family backgrounds; adaptability; sexuality; intimacy; stress management; children; and chores and leisure activities, some of which have already been dealt with at the beginning of their relationship.

Racial and cultural differences can also challenge societal messages about marriage within one's culture. Within a culturally homogenous model of marriage (same race/culture), people are assumed to have similar racial and cultural backgrounds and therefore have similar instructions and messages of how to deal with culture and race within their relationship, but that is also seldom completely the case. Within a culturally heterogeneous marriage (interracial/intercultural), partners must in some way negotiate and accommodate these differences. Does one person's culture take precedence over the other, leaving one culture invisible? How do those with culturally heterogeneous marriages work out these complexities? Although differences in race and culture can make the construction of shared meaning in marriage an area of negotiation, it is unclear to what extent such challenges are automatic or simply related to something else.

How Do We as Clinicians Address This?

Understanding the realities and co-construction of those in interracial relationships is crucial to understanding their experiences, formed through their relationships with each other, others, and various contexts. Thus, clinicians must attend to the variety of contexts and relationships that inform the couple's relationship. These truths are constructed through understandings of meanings of age, gender, education, sexuality, culture, etc., which influence each person's identity and form the links to society (Burr, 2003). Through dominant meaning-making and an organized effort of maintenance, society has what may seem to be an inexorable and irremovable power on an individual. Clinicians should be aware and curious about how partners successfully manage their meaning as a couple through societal power.

Ecological Systems Theory

Couples must navigate a variety of systems of relationships throughout their lifetimes, as well as daily. To further expand nuances of couple meaning and interaction within a larger social context, we use Bronfenbrenner's (1986) ecological systems theory. This theory aims to understand an individual's life and daily process; however, we use his theory to conceptually organize how multiple relationships with environments from various social contexts, systems, and levels impact a couple. Bronfenbrenner's ecological systems theory (1986) integrates five systemic levels of interaction: microsystem, mesosystem, exosystem, macrosystem, and chronosystem.

For an interracial and intercultural couple, the microsystem refers to each individual within the couple dyad. Examining this level will enable an inside look at the beliefs and attitudes of each partner shaped from previous and current relationships that help shape their couple identity and the meaning of being in an interracial relationship. Specific shared experiences that shape the couple will also be addressed at this level. For example, one would want to understand the meaning and beliefs that partners attribute to specific co-created traditions and how that shapes their relationship after experiencing these themes together.

The environmental influences and interactions as a couple—through their relationships with home, work, and school—encompass the mesosystem (Bronfenbrenner, 1986). At this level, the focus will be directed to influences from and interactions with families of origin, friendships, and other relationships. For example, addressing this level would emphasize the attitudes from the families of origin in response to the choice of an interracial relationship and how that shapes the couple.

The exosystem, for an interracial couple, includes community influences, which could extend from their neighborhood or religious communities to larger social systems, such as the media, laws, and societal norms—For example, recent media headlines of the Roe vs Wade overturn raised concern and questions around current federal protection (or lack thereof at the time) for interracial and same-sex marriage in the United States (Ciesemier & Goodwin, 2022; The Associated Press, 2022). For an interracial couple, these can be a source of disconnect or support between partners. There may be a sense of instability overall, as the couple must become aware of shared cultural values, beliefs, customs, and laws across other races and ethnicities that can serve as advocacy (i.e., The Federal Defense of Marriage Act). The macrosystem impacts the couple through societal attitudes and conceptualizations about interracial couples. For example, the legalization of interracial marriage initiated the beginning of the acceptance of interracial couple relationships; yet others due to macro influences have still been influenced by the old ways of thinking. Within the macrosystem, messages from culture, race, ethnicity, and marriage are also an influence, which filter through bias. Lastly, the chronosystem refers to time and nodal transitions and events for an individual. This does not include global history and time; this would be better addressed by the macrosystem (Bronfenbrenner, 1986). For an interracial couple, this could refer to the loss of family following marriage if the family is not supportive.

By addressing how a couple navigates these five levels, one can systemically understand a couple's process relationally, which penetrates below-surface issues (i.e., process vs. content). Utilizing ecological systems theory enables understanding an interracial couple from a variety of stances to gain a holistic perspective and make visible daily realities from significant relationships in their worlds (family, community, and society). With this holistic perspective, a better understanding can be gained regarding how interracial couples create strong and meaningful relationships to navigate their world as a couple, relationships with others, and within society.

An Important Note of Consideration

The term "interracial" is often used interchangeably with intercultural and interethnic and is sometimes referred to as intermarried or intermixing (Seshadri & Knudson-Martin, 2013). Race and ethnicity are often intermixed as well. For example, Hispanic (descendants from Spanish-speaking populations) and Latino/a/e/x (descendants from Latin America) categorizations are used interchangeably with race and ethnicity but are referred to as ethnicity rather than race in the census in 2010, which is filtered within the literature depending on when it was published (United States Census Bureau, 2010). Although their definitions are considered different, many researchers also interchange "interracial" and "intercultural" with terms such as "interethnic," "intermarried," "heterogamy," and "intermixing." Brooks (2022), in a metanalytic review, even found publication bias with finding those doing interracial research (i.e., smaller sample sizes) in comparison with those with intraracial relationships (i.e., larger sample sizes). Results demonstrated that comparing satisfaction levels in interracial relationships was flawed due to incomparable sample sizes and availability of access.

Consistent with a social constructionist perspective, it is important to note that society's perceptions of race and how to make meaning of difference is changing. In contrast to the 2000 United States Census, which denoted race as including only five categories—Asian, White, Native American, Pacific Islander, and Black—with no room for other ethnic variations (i.e., Indian, Hispanic, Middle Eastern, etc.), beginning with the 2010 census, the form included many different possible racial and ethnic intersections and enabled a person to select more than one category and/or define their own racial/ethnic description; this was the first time this was permitted to be categorized (United States Census Bureau, 2010). In 2020, the census became further diversified including two separate questions, one for race and one for Hispanic or Latino origin (United States Census Bureau, 2021). It has been suggested that the 2020 census demonstrated that people are more diverse than was anticipated due to people's multiracial and ethnic heritages. It is not surprising that the conceptualization of interracial and/or intercultural couples becomes confused.

Overview of This Book

In the following chapters, we will explore relevant life cycles and how a mental health professional can help interracial, intercultural, and interfaith couples and families navigate them. Thus far, in this first chapter, we have given a brief description of the need to understand interracial, intercultural, and interfaith experiences and the frameworks we will be using, social constructionism and ecological systems theory. Next, we will introduce our social locations and discuss the importance of intersectionality. Chapter 2 addresses the importance of the self of the therapist in relationship to interracial and intercultural partners, especially in the areas of bias. Chapter 3 discusses interracial and intercultural attraction and how this may influence a couple at this life stage. Chapter 4 focuses on how a couple can start to negotiate their differences while having to deal with multiple systems, family, friends, community, etc., among race and culture. Chapter 5 explores how cohabitation might impact these couples and key areas for therapists to pay attention to. Chapter 6 considers how marriage, children, blended families, religion/spirituality, and non-monogamy can be influenced by interracial, intercultural, and interfaith issues. Chapter 7 analyzes how racial and cultural dynamics influence retirement, legacy, and expectations. Chapter 8 discusses hot-button topics: Sex, politics, and religion, with an afterword for the book. The appendix after each chapter incorporates suggested exercises for mental health professionals based on the previous chapters to extend practice and knowledge.

Intersectionality Framework

We believe that one cannot discuss race, culture, religion/spirituality, and ethnicity within the interracial couple and family experience without discussing intersectionality. Intersectionality refers to the multidimensionality of social identities (i.e., race, ethnicity, sexual orientation, gender, and ability) and how experiences of bias, discrimination, inequity, and identity construction and maintenance are based on societal advantage and disadvantage. By contextualizing converging points of power and disadvantage, intersectionality invites further exploration of the experiences of interracial couples and families to uncover hierarchical systems of domination and subordination, as well as the understanding of the power supporting the dynamic between differing cultural identities and intersecting systems of inequality (Crenshaw, 1991). An intersectional lens also helps expand the focus of this book beyond cisgender, heterosexual relationships, all including a wider range of sexual orientations, gender identities, etc. We also want to be explicit that we are intentionally using both the terms couple and partners, as couples can suggest a binary lens. Further, we also use the word "family" or "partners" in the non-monogamy section instead of couple.

We invite readers to think about couples and families with the Hays' ADDRESSING model (i.e., age, disability, religion, ethnicity, socioeconomic status, sexual orientation, indigenous heritage, national origin, and gender). According to Hays, integrating this approach provides clinicians and researchers a framework for understanding underrepresented groups and oppressive forces, as we explore the complexities of intersecting identities in psychology and relationships. Couples who occupy multiple social locations may also experience discrepancies between privilege and disadvantage that they will inevitably need to negotiate between themselves and others, and which needs to be validated and addressed by mental health professionals and each other. Lastly, while most previous research has been focused on heterosexual, cisgender, nonimmigrant/citizens, able-bodied, intrareligious, educated, middle-class or upper-middle-class, interracial couples, we encourage readers to use this book and intersectional framework with those who don't embody these social locations and modify as appropriate, with thoughtful reflection and insight.

Author Introductions

Gita Seshadri (she/her). I am a youthful-in-appearance, South Asian American, middle-class/educated, able-bodied, heterosexual female, with a chronic illness, in an interracial, intercultural, and interfaith relationship with a multiracial (White and Asian), cisgender, heterosexual man. I have intersections of both privilege and disadvantage and am mindful of this and how I negotiate differences with him throughout our relationship. Advocacy and understanding of interracial relationships have long been a passion of mine, both clinically and through research; I bring humility, intersectionality, and an openness to learning.

Dumayi Gutierrez (she/her). I identify as AfroLatina, cisfemale with femme expression, lesbian, able-bodied, with upper-middle-class privileges. I am also in an interracial marriage with a White, lesbian, cisgender female, with androgynous expression, and we are parents to two multiracial daughters. I have always had a passion for working with BIPOC LGBTQ+ communities and intersectional culturally humble approaches. In all aspects of my life, I seek to embody intersectionality, empowerment, and social justice; yet I always have so much to learn.

Our Invitation

As our reader, we invite you as a clinician to consider our insights based on our professional and clinical work over the last two decades in treating interracial, intercultural, and interfaith relationships and families. Please note, all chapter and clinical examples and case applications have been modified to protect confidentiality for all. Any resemblances to specific individuals or couples are purely coincidental. Let us show you what we have learned.

References

Berger, P., & Kellner, H. (1994). Marriage and the construction of reality: An exercise in the microsociology of knowledge. In G. Handel & G. G. Whitchurch (Eds.), *The psychosocial interior of the family* (4th ed., pp. 19–36). Aldine de Gruyter.

Bratter, J. L., & Eschbach, K. (2006). What about the couple? Interracial marriage and psychological distress. *Social Science Research, 35*(4), 1025–1047.

Bratter, J. L., & King, R. B. (2008). "But will it last?": Marital instability among interracial and same-race-couples. *Family Relations, 57*(2), 160–171. https://doi.org/10.1016/j.ssresearch.2005.09.001

Bronfenbrenner, U. (1986). Ecology of the family as a context for human development: Research perspectives. *Developmental Psychology, 22*, 723–742. https://doi.org/10.1037/0012-1649.22.6.723

Brooks, J. (2022). Differences in satisfaction? A meta-analytic review of interracial and intraracial relationships. *Marriage & Family Review, 58*(2), 129–157. https://doi.org/10.1080/01494929.2021.1937443

Brown, C. C., Williams, Z., & Durtschi, J. A. (2018). Trajectories of interracial heterosexual couples: A longitudinal analysis of relationship quality and separation. *Journal of Marital and Family Therapy, 45*, 650–667. https://doi.org/10.1111/jmft.12363

Buggs, S. G. (2019). Color, culture, or cousin? Multiracial Americans and framing boundaries in interracial relationships. *Journal of Marriage and Family, 81*(5), 1221–1236. https://doi.org/10.1111/jomf.12583

Burr, V. (2003). *Social constructionism* (2nd ed.). Routledge.

Childs, E. (2004). *Interracial images: Popular culture depictions of Black-White couples.* American Sociological Association annual meeting 2004, San Francisco, CA.

Ciesemier, K., & Goodwin, M. (Hosts). (2022, June 9). How dismantling Roe puts interracial marriage at risk [Audio podcast episode]. In *Liberty Podcast*. ACLU. https://www.aclu.org/podcast/how-dismantling-roe-puts-interracial-marriage-at-risk

Collins, P. H. (2000). Gender, Black feminism, and Black political economy. *The Annals of the American Academy of Political and Social Science, 568*(1), 41–53. https://doi.org/10.1177/000271620056800105

Crenshaw, K. (1991). Mapping the margins: Intersectionality, identity politics, and violence against Women of Color. *Stanford Law Review, 43*(6), 1241–1299. https://doi.org/10.2307/1229039

Fu, X., Tora, J., & Kendall, H. (2001). Marital happiness and inter-racial marriage: A briefing in a multi-ethnic community in Hawaii. *Journal of Comparative Family Studies, 32*(1), 47–60. https://doi.org/10.3138/jcfs.32.1.47

Gergen, K. (2015). Horizons of human inquiry. In *An invitation to social construction* (3rd ed., pp. 61–89). SAGE. https://doi.org/10.4135/9781473921276

Han, B. (2021). Race, gender, and power in Asian American interracial marriages. *Social Science Research, 96*, 102542. https://doi.org/10.1016/j.ssresearch.2021.102542

Hibbler, D., & Shinew, K. J. (2002). Interracial couples' experience of leisure: A social network approach. *Journal of Leisure Research, 34*(2), 135–157. https://doi.org/10.1080/00222216.2002.11949966

Killian, K. D. (2002). Dominant and marginalized discourses in interracial couples' narratives: Implications for family therapists. *Family Process, 41*, 603–619. https://doi.org/10.1111/j.1545-5300.2002.00603.x

Killian, K. D. (2003). Homogamy outlaws: Interracial couples' strategic responses to racism and to partner differences. In V. Thomas, T. A. Karis, & J. L. Wetchler (Eds.), *Clinical issues with interracial couples: Theories and research* (pp. 3–21). Hawthorne Press.

Lewandowski, D. A., & Jackson, L. A. (2001). Perceptions of interracial couples: Prejudice at the dyadic level. *Journal of Black Psychology, 27*(3), 288–303. https://doi.org/10.1177/0095798401027003003

Livingston, G. (2017, May 18). *99 percent of all marriages were intrarracial in 1970, as of 2015, the number has decreased to 83 percent.* Pew Research Center. http://www.pewresearch.org/fact-tank/2017/05/18/in-u-s-metro-areas-huge-variationin-intermarriage-rates/

MCarthy, J. (2021, September 10). *U.S. approval of interracial marriage at new high of 94%.* Gallup. https://news.gallup.com/poll/354638/approval-interracial-marriage-new-high.aspx

Mills, J., & Daly, J. (1995). A note on family acceptance involving interracial friendships and romantic relationships. *Journal of Psychology, 129*(3), 349–352.

Nemoto, K. (2004). *Race still matters: Popular discourse of interracial marriage and Asian American experiences* [Conference paper]. American Sociological Association annual meeting 2004, San Francisco, CA.

Paré, D. A. (1996). Culture and meaning: Expanding the metaphorical repertoire of family therapy. *Family Process, 35*(1), 21–42. https://doi.org/10.1111/j.1545-5300.1996.00021.x

Parker, K., & Barroso, A. (2021, February 25). *In vice president Kamala Harris, we can see how America has changed.* Pew Research Center. https://policycommons.net/artifacts/1426333/in-vice-president-kamala-harris-we-can-see-how-america-has-changed/2040752/

Schueths, A. M. (2014). 'It's almost like White supremacy': Interracial mixed-status couples facing racist nativism. *Ethnic & Racial Studies, 37*(13), 2438–2456. https://doi.org/10.1080/01419870.2013.835058

Seshadri, G., & Knudson-Martin, C. (2013). How couples manage interracial and intercultural differences: Implications for clinical practice. *Journal of Marital and Family Therapy, 39*, 43–58. https://doi.org/10.1111/j.1752-0606.2011.00262.x

Shankar, P. R., & Subish, P. (2016). Fair skin in South Asia: An obsession? *Journal of Pakistan Association of Dermatology, 17*(2), 100–104. https://jpad.com.pk/index.php/jpad/article/viewFile/695/668

Solsberry, P. W. (1994). Interracial couples in The United States of America: Implications for mental health counseling. *Journal of Mental Health Counseling, 16*(3), 304–318.

Steinbugler, A. C. (2005). Visibility as privilege and danger: Heterosexual and same-sex interracial intimacy in the 21st century. *Sexualities, 8*(4), 425–443. https://doi.org/10.1177/1363460705056618

Sullivan, R. (2005). *What about the children? Black/White children, family approval of interracial relationships, and contemporary racial ideology.* Annual meeting of the American Sociological Association annual meeting, Philadelphia, PA.

The Associated Press. (2022, July 19). *Bill to protect same-sex and interracial marriage passes overwhelmingly in the House.* NPR Politics. https://www.npr.org/2022/07/19/1112213293/house-vote-same-sex-marriage

Thompson, J., & Collier, M. J. (2006). Toward contingent understandings of intersecting identifications among selected U.S. interracial couples: Integrating interpretive and critical views. *Communication Quarterly, 54*(4), 487–506. https://doi.org/10.1080/01463370601036671

U.S. Census Bureau. (2010). *Overview of race and Hispanic Origin:2010.* The Census Bureau: 2010 Census Briefs. https://www.census.gov/content/dam/Census/library/publications/2011/dec/c2010br-02.pdf

U.S. Census Bureau. (2018, July 9). *Growth in interracial and interethnic married-couple households.* The Census Bureau: Race, Ethnicity, and Marriage in the United States. https://www.census.gov/library/stories/2018/07/interracial-marriages.html

U.S. Census Bureau. (2021, August 12). *2020 census illuminates racial and ethnic composition of the country.* United States Census Bureau: Improved race and ethnicity measures reveal U.S. population is much more multiracial. https://www.census.gov/library/stories/2018/07/interracial-marriages.html

Chapter 2
Who Am I? Who Are You? Self of the Therapist Exploration

"I am me. In all the world, there is no one else exactly like me. Everything that comes out of me is authentically mine, because I alone chose it." Virginia Satir

Satir (1995)

As mental health professionals, using ourselves in therapy is often viewed as second nature; as our clients are in the room, so are we. Many have acknowledged the importance of exploration of self through common factors, role of therapist in different theories, and even countertransference; however continual questions arise as to how "the self" can be used with social elements and context (Aponte, 2022; Aponte & Kissil, 2016). Bringing in oneself has often been seen as harmful and to be avoided under the guise of needing to maintain objectivity (Aponte, 2022). Graduate programs in marriage and family therapy emphasize the use of self in therapy but often don't go beyond the abstract; there is limited demonstration of practice, much less with interracial and intercultural couples.

Aponte (2022) encouraged therapists to use the person of the therapist model, where he alluded to using the self as an avenue of empathy and connection to clients. By selectively and purposefully connecting with a client through the therapist's vulnerability, the client can have the experiential experience of empathy. When considering interracial and intercultural partnering, the self of the therapist plays a key role in treatment because this process of empathy and sociocultural attunement can be fraught with difficulty. For example, a therapist might privately say to themselves that they would never choose interracial partnering because their family would never allow it, or avoid it as an option with a biased lens (e.g., saying consciously or unconsciously, "I *would* date interracially/interculturally, but I am only attracted to people with (stereotyped preferences), or I don't have interaction with groups outside of my race, etc."). The therapist may also promote "collaboration" while ignoring culture and using a one-size-fits-all approach (e.g., one partner must reject their culture for the sake of their partner's culture, or focusing only on

© American Family Therapy Academy (AFTA) 2024

G. Seshadri, D. Gutierrez, *Interracial, Intercultural, and Interfaith Couples and Families Across the Life Cycle*, AFTA SpringerBriefs in Family Therapy, https://doi.org/10.1007/978-3-031-58538-8_2

broad issues like communication, trust, etc.). Direct experience is not demanded for empathy; rather, an integration of self, culture, and client is required. Thus, we use a multicultural self of the therapist model when looking at interracial and intercultural partners. If we don't, we risk missing something about our interracial, intercultural, or interreligious clients—or worse, harm them with our ignorance.

Insight and Microsystem Influences on Self of the Therapist

Therapists are important for conveying hope and warmth during therapy; we believe in our clients and can hold our clients' painful experiences. Being mindful of the therapist's role and presence, therapists must explore their experiences of power struggles within the family, parental conflicts, lack of validation, and lack of intimacy in relationships. Therapists often work multifacetedly, navigating intrapersonal wholeness; mind, body, and emotional integration; communication; authenticity; and recognition of self, individuals, couples, families, and larger systems. For example, influences and attitudes from family of origin (mesosystem) and implicit rules of "not marrying outside race or ethnicity" or "partner has to meet cultural expectations in a spouse" may contribute to a heightened expectation of the "perfect" relationship. In taking on the task of self of the therapist work, the therapist can deconstruct rigidity through personal awareness developed through self-reflection or personal therapy to promote flexibility with their clients. While both the Interracial Couple Questionnaire and the Multiple Heritage Questionnaire help the therapist to start this work, there must be a deeper dive (Henriksen et al., 2007; Watts & Henriksen, 1998).

Meso- and Exosystem Influences in Self-Disclosure

The practice of self-disclosure is commonly associated with therapists bringing the self into therapeutic processes during sessions with their client(s). Although it has origins in psychoanalysis, self-disclosure has evolved into an appropriate way to establish trust with the client, instead of relying primarily on tone, eye contact, and body language. Since interracial couples and families may already experience oppression accompanied by feelings such as loneliness and isolation, the connection offered by self-disclosure may help to allay these emotions and be an avenue of empathy. For example, a therapist in a same-sex interracial marriage may resonate with or have similar experiences of their clients with similar social location of navigating sexuality, race, and gender. This type of sharing is increasingly helpful in working with BIPOC clients to develop trust. However, when self-disclosure is offered in a biased way, it becomes problematic (Dansby Olufowote et al., 2022) and can also be seen as crossing a boundary (Psychopathology Committee, 2001). For example, this can happen if the therapist over-identifies with the client of color or the client of majority culture, or misinterprets cultural rules or traditions based on their own lack of understanding or experiences. Without self-awareness, therapists could easily make mistakes. Adding to the example, this therapist may have experienced a tremulous coming out experience and learned to cope via avoidance, which may vastly differ from their clients' experience. In aligning with the negative experiences of the couple and their own coping mechanisms, the therapist may miss the joys and resiliencies around sexuality and ethnicity.

Self-disclosure during work with clients in interracial and intercultural relationships is rarely discussed, let alone how a therapist can navigate their own biases. This may be due to fears around these discussions and discomfort with acknowledging judgements or biases; in therapy, the "rule" is that we as professionals are nonjudgmental. The fear is often translated from not wanting to be viewed as racist, sexist, phobic, etc., and therefore, these topics are avoided by being smoothed over immediately.

Professional ethics and learning institutions often require therapists to be culturally competent (knowledge and education) and sensitive (awareness of cultures); while that is helpful, being culturally humble (the acknowledgment that we will never fully understand another culture's experience) (Hsieh & Quek, 2021) is required. In essence, sensitivity and competency, are an awareness of cultures different than our own and building knowledge of cultural values, and not tokenizing the minority group/class with any type of intersectionality (i.e., race, gender, ethnicity, socioeconomic status, and religion) by expecting them to teach us instead. Humility suggests therapists engage in continual self-exploration and considers this paramount to being clinically active.

On-going self-exploration is often not employed for a variety of reasons, leaving therapists to metaphorically check the box and feel "certified" that they practice cultural humility and are free from having to continually engage in this process. Again, the block may also arise due to feeling that as therapists, they are inherently nonjudgmental in their practice, once they have been seasoned in the field for a few years, or even after they have taken their diversity course within their graduate program. The pressure of being perceived as role models can create an environment where the therapist feels that with all they have learned, they have *arrived* professionally, through a sense of entitlement. Sometimes, this process takes the opposite direction, with imposture syndrome, where despite high achieving abilities, the therapist in some ways feels like a fraud and questions their professional mindset. Thus, they may seek to act knowledgeably and lead with this rather than with humility or empathy, or take a distant objective stance to hide their feelings of incompetence.

Lastly, mental health professionals by default must interact with organizations and professional entities where judgement is key; the process of diagnosing and using the medical model inherently asks mental health professionals to "judge" clients; we are simply asking them to continue to exercise their awareness more humbly in these aspects. To work with interracial and intercultural partners, therapists don't just need to know about their self of the therapist issues with each person's specific culture; they also may need to know how to help the couple negotiate differences around their cultural traditions, values, and practices. Moreover, "the best therapist directories" seldom list work with interracial, intercultural, or interfaith couples/families as part of their presenting issues and leave an overall category of "racial identity" work, which further marginalizes these oppressed groups and makes the process more arduous for both the clients and the therapist (Dansby Olufowote et al., 2022).

Positionality (Micro-, Meso-, Exo-, and Macrosystem Influences)

Clinicians in training learn that couples navigate subjectivity in their world based on their intrapersonal selves, interpersonal relationships, and influential systems related to their environments (e.g., society, culture, work setting, and neighborhood). They also learn that our personal and professional experiences influence our theoretical orientations, perceptions of problems, and presence. Integration of our experiences into therapy is a "parallel process," an interaction between clients and therapists that replicates patterns of behavior and language, which contributes to therapeutic alliance and human connection (Gutierrez, 2018). For example, a client may be struggling to meet the romantic needs of their partner. Simultaneously, the therapist, also in a romantic relationship, may be experiencing the same issue in their life. Rather than the therapist becoming overly intertwined in their client experience (e.g., countertransference), there is an openness to reflect on both of their processes. The therapist takes the opportunity to explore how they are similar, different, human, etc. and pay attention to work through this issue. Thus, the therapist is not only guiding the client in their experience but is taking in and collaborating with them while processing their own.

When working with interracial and intercultural couples, therapists' subjective experiences come through parallel processes; our positionality and social locations become crucial to recognizing power, oppression, and cultural sensitivity in the therapy session. A starting place for clinicians to investigate their cultural heritage, privilege, and navigation within a sociocultural context is the ADDRESSING model (Hays, 2001). This model says we have a duty to ourselves and our clients to be aware of and express our social locations, including age, developmental and acquired abilities, sexual orientation, socioeconomic status, gender, sex, national origin, religion, ethnic and racial identities, etc. Essentially, we are responsible for understanding the identities and constructs that drive and navigate us throughout our lives.

Through our clinical training, most of us have completed genograms and assignments on our families of origin to increase our self-awareness. However, examining our identities and working within parallel processes shouldn't stop here. Building from Hay's ADDRESSING model, Hardy (2018) proposed the need to reflect on implicit and explicit intergenerational beliefs that have shaped us and informed our realities. These beliefs are based on societal scripts, "implicit expectations that individuals develop to understand and deal with emotionally significant life experiences" (Demorest, 2013, p. 583), directing us how we are expected to behave and feel. As explicit rules align relationships and families regarding finances, chores, consequences, etc.; implicit rules drive behavior considered socially desirable. For example (implicitly), individuals may believe that their personalities were naturally created; others believe their personalities are shaped and developed over time (Franuik et al., 2002). Regarding romantic relationships, some individuals may expect to find their soulmate and to be passionately in love, while others may expect the relationship to unfold as it is, believing that perfect compatibility doesn't exist (Franuik et al., 2002). In both cases, these beliefs created values and biases that are invisible until the clinician can make them visible to themselves.

Further, our own intersectionalities reflect these implicit and explicit intergenerational beliefs. For example, a White heterosexual, cisgender therapist is working with a heterosexual, interracial couple including a Black cisgender man (Damien) and a White cisgender woman (Amy), and during one session they are discussing Black Lives Matter (BLM) movement in the United States. Growing up in a strong, Black family, with open discussions of race, Damien may implicitly expect Amy to recognize BLM's impact on their lives (e.g., she will honor the struggles of my family and prior generations. She will be sure to engage with me in the social justice of our communities. How could she not think about these issues in this way? Or how could she not consider how I feel about this or expect me to not personalize this?). However, both Amy and the therapist, growing up in families of privileged status regarding race (not needing to think about this), may have limited exposure to discussions about race or social justice and don't understand the need to continually discuss racial issues or how this can be personal to Damien.

In session, Amy is seen as looking away/looking down, or even deflecting the conversation back to other relational issues. In this dynamic, Damien becomes increasingly upset that Amy does not understand the severity of his fears as a Black man driving in their city, and Amy shows signs of withdrawing to cope with heightened emotions. In seeing their dynamic, the therapist may work to decrease their tension and work on their communication styles. However, the therapist can miss a necessary dialogue on race, power, and how to navigate their feelings as a couple, or even a couple in society. Further, in doing so, the therapist might subtly create a coalition with Amy around race because they are not seeing the deeper meaning of how race is personal to Damien and his family of origin and inadvertently privileging the choice (i.e., the option to avoid) to not have the conversation even further. This would be based upon the White therapist or the White partner knowing that Black people (and their partner) face injustice but not empathically feeling or resonating with that experience. The role of the therapist would be to facilitate emotional attunement and connection around this topic so that tension wouldn't increase between the couple and the therapist, and they all could move out of the dynamics of privilege and oppression playing out in the session.

For therapist development, active awareness of their own identity development is needed to process and make sense of these reactions. Exploring power and identity intersections, social location, and sociocultural factors increases our cultural humility and attunement to the various cultures present in our therapy rooms. Shared social identities do not recuse the therapeutic relationship from cultural mishaps, microaggressions, navigation of space, or disproportionate power roles (Jernigan et al., 2010). As observers, multidirectional beings, and systems thinkers, couple and family therapists can envision the simultaneous intersections of culture and multiple relational processes.

Using the example of Damien and Amy having a discussion around race and taking a stance of cultural humility, the therapist could facilitate a discussion around helping Amy hear and show empathy and understanding around the impact of BLM, race, and family of origin in terms of legacy, using this as a point of connection, instead of having Damien teach both about his culture. In this way, Damien does not become of token, needing to continually teach others about his experiences as a minority Black male. In addition, using intersectionality, the therapist could help Amy use her voice as a female within this relationship while managing Amy's anxiety around these discussions.

Cultural Responsiveness

Working within an intersectional and culturally responsive perspective involves the therapist's ability to step back and step out of an encapsulated worldview. Encapsulation is when therapists maintain their own implicit and explicit beliefs, imposing them onto clients, rather than providing a collaborative space and advocating for the client's cultural narratives (Bergkamp & Ponsford, 2020). Movement away from encapsulation involves a continuum of the therapist's awareness and cultural journey throughout their professional careers. Continuing this journey is the essence of culturally responsive work not only for general practice as a mental health clinician but is also imperative in working with interracial and intercultural clients. Literature has shown that culturally responsive therapy involves epistemological theories (e.g., social constructionism, feminism, critical race theory), attention to context (sociopolitical, sociocultural, intersectional systems, historical context), attention to culture (tradition, values, worldview, experiences), methodology (attention to intersectionality, client-centered, nontraditional measures and measures designed to fit with diverse populations), collaboration (clients and families, community members, therapist and supervisors, advisors boards, cultural advocates, accountability structures), and a movement past pathologizing (empowerment, critique and criticism to dominant power structures, and movement away from generalization) (Seponski et al., 2013, pp. 29–30).

Another example on a macro level might be looked at like this: a therapist was living during a time when racism, sexism, etc. was particularly high and discrimination was blatant. Self-work would involve challenging one's own biases and exploring how the family triggers these, not to mention societal messages around race relations and community experiences. Furthermore, utilizing supervision and/ or consultation is essential to promote continual culturally responsive growth, self-awareness, and self of the therapist work.

Development of contextual self-awareness is a continual process that is not linear. As a part of self-exploration, self of the therapist, and intersectionality, we invite clinicians to explore their professional identity further by addressing their own journeys by revisiting ecological systems theory and social construction. Previously, Chap. 1 gave summaries of social construction, ecological systems theory, and systems theory.

Ecological Systems Theory and Self of the Therapist

Here we revisit Seshadri and Knudson's (2013) application of Bronfenbrenner's ecological systems theory (1986), in which the couple was the central microsystem to show how the therapist may interact with each level (See Table 2.1 and Appendix 2.1). What follows from the original model (Seshadri & Knudson-Martin, 2013) are the questions that the clinician may ask themselves when engaging in self of the therapist work in relationship with their client couple or family.

For therapists, looking at their role within the "we" is paramount. For example, if the therapist has the same ethnic background as one of the interracial partners, this clinician will have to explore how their identities and experiences could be different from that partner. Does it make a difference that the clinician and the partner are different in their intersectionality; what if they were the same?

Using the example of Damien and Amy, the therapist would have to question how they have responded to racial issues in the past within themselves; let's say that the therapist believes in equality, but at times doesn't see the need to have conversations about race "in everything." The therapist must challenge themselves to step outside of ways they are previously used to being, for the sake of the client (microsystem). Continuing the example, if the therapist does some deep reflection and realizes that this need to not "include race in everything" stems from comments that their parents made while growing up that were biased (mesosystem) and missed opportunities that they felt they didn't have, such as job promotions, scholarships, etc. (mesosystem/exosystem). Further, the therapist may realize that having these conversations may indirectly touch upon the therapist's belief that perhaps there is still continual work that needs to be done to address racism (macrosystem). How they deal with this over time and if they continue to see interracial, intercultural, and/or interreligious partners or families determines how they integrate these processes (chronosystem).

Table 2.1 Application of ecological systems theory and self of the therapist

Microsystem: Creating the "We": Influences inside the couple/partners relationship that shape their identity, strength, and meaning. This includes each individual's perceived realities	The therapist's identities, alliance, and influence impact the interracial/intercultural couple/partner dyad: Questions: How do my identities/social locations (ADDRESSING), influence the interracial partners (my clients)? Would I ever choose an interracial relationship or not? Why or why not? What biases/self-reflection have led me to this? (avoidance or intentional choice)
Mesosystem: We and Us: The couple/partners and their experiences with current or previous friends and family in relationship to them	The therapist's experiences and meanings with their own families and friends impact the interracial/intercultural couple/partner dyad: Questions: How do my current and previous friends and family influence the work with the interracial couple/partners? What biases (positive or negative) do I have about culture, race, religion from growing up (related to humor, specific events, trauma, etc.) How might these experiences influence what I highlight/use as interventions in the context of the therapy room?
Exosystem: We and Them: The couple/partners and their interactions with their own communities and cultures in relationship to the therapist	Therapist's communities of influence and experiences and the meanings of their own culture and other cultures impact the interracial/intercultural couple/partner dyad: Questions: How does my community(ies) and culture(s) work with the interracial couple/partners? Are there any cultural or racial or religious tensions or bias? How will I manage this in the room and within myself? What previous communities have I been a part of that may influence me (humor, specific events, trauma, etc.)
Macrosystem: We and the World: The couple/partners and their interactions with society/social media/media, government, culture, race, gender, society at large, advocacy in relationship to the therapist	The therapist's experiences and meanings—how does my view of society, social media, government, culture, race, gender, and society at large impact the interracial/intercultural couple/partner dyad: Questions: What do I think about the government, its influence, and its social policies? What do I think of current social issues and how they may impact interracial/intercultural couples? What are my feelings about advocacy and how it's currently being carried out right now in relation to race, culture, and/or religion?

(continued)

Table 2.1 (continued)

Chronosystem: We and Life: The couple/partners and their interactions with time and pivotal events in relationship with the therapist and the progress of treatment	The therapist's own personal experiences, biases, opinions, and countertransference: Questions: How do time, events, and my personal experiences, biases, and countertransference influence the work with the interracial couple/partners? /How do I express my humility? How am I making progress through my self-work? How will this impact my empathy over time and burnout? Am I changing my opinions through my continual work after self-reflection? What am I doing differently?

Extended Reflection

Through self of the therapist work, therapists would have to look at their families of origin and how they might interact with interracial, intercultural, and interfaith pairings. Would there be jokes, rejection, or social ostracization? Even small jokes can suggest bias from the present or even early experiences. Therapists need to ask themselves how these systems have shaped them and how they are currently shaping them. When exploring community, common cultural practices come into question. For example, attending plantation parties (common occurrences or pastimes in the South as a part of tradition) or even the use of the N word in songs, which are repeated when either lip-synching, or singing the song becomes questionable when exploring the community influences of the therapist. For example, how are they integrating these experiences? Are they viewing it as a part of history that they are no longer connected to? What are the implications of these behaviors? This way of thinking and reflection helps therapists explore how the larger social systems they participate in influence them.

Perceptions and experiences around laws and the government can play a role as well for the therapist. For example, stances on immigration, or even being affected by other laws around categorization (i.e., the census), can all filter into therapeutic work indirectly.

Lastly, clinicians need to think of times in their own lives when personal experiences, bias, played a role across time. Like, if a therapist was cut off from their own sibling due to their sibling's choice of being in an interracial, intercultural, or interfaith pairing and how the sibling did or did not communicate this to the family. Appendix 2.1 offers a graphical representation of how this can impact both the couple/family and the therapist along with additional questions for extended reflective exercises.

Case Application

When Frank (Latinx, heterosexual, cisgender male, masculine expression) and Susie (Multiethnic American, heterosexual, cisgender female, feminine expression) came to therapy, it became clear after a few sessions that they needed to work on integrating their cultures, families, and experiences into their relationship to strengthen their parental subsystem and marriage. Following several sessions, it was evident that they were on the battlefield against each other, rather than working together on the same side. Frank exhibited the need to lead and protect his family, often booming with a loud voice when discussing his narrative. His positionality would be open-chested, wide-legged, and forward, sitting almost off the couch. Susie exhibited independence and a need to bring calmness/direction to her family. She leaned back into the couch, open-chested, chin up, often with arms crossed listening to her husband's booming voice, waiting for him to stop so she could share her perspective; many times, she needed to introject.

With both being alpha, dominant, and you as a 5'2", small-framed therapist, their positionality as a couple was physically and metaphorically dominant in the therapy room. To be honest, it made you sweat! Through the sweat, you experienced a dual interactive process of connecting to intergenerational, cultural structures while resonating with navigation of gender and ethnicity. Despite all being People of Color (POC) in the room, there is a struggle for power and space.

Maintaining your self of the therapist work involved awareness of paralleling Susie's role as a Women of Color (WOC) and Frank's Latinx culture, while maintaining curiosity about their dominance (pure strength they exuded as a couple, powerful when they turned on one another). Will you feel vulnerable at times? Yes, but that was "humanness" coming into the room. Through your own identity development, you realize that you are holding an internalized expectation; correlating power to space when the goal was to reframe empowerment through curiosity and growth. It was a reminder to model congruency and calmness for them through sitting back in the chair, taking deep breaths, and creating a safe space for healing. Eventually, the battlefield went from opposing sides to allies.

Lessons from the Chapter

In this chapter, we discussed the potential sources and influences of biases across ecological systems and direct application to working with interracial, intercultural, and interfaith couples. We highlighted the importance of cultural humility, self-awareness, and practicing this across one's professional career. Continual ways to exercise self-reflection are encouraged.

Appendix 2.1: The Self of the Therapist and the Interracial/Intercultural/Interfaith Partners

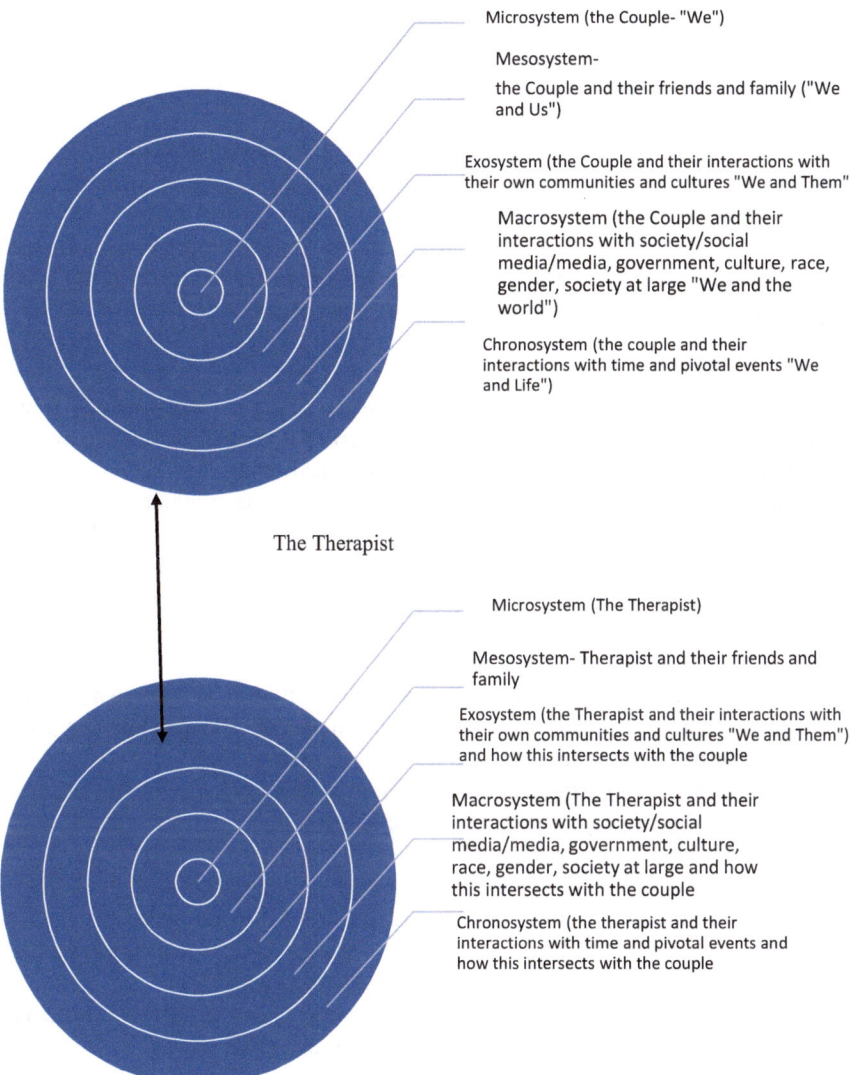

Microsystem (the Couple- "We")

Mesosystem-
the Couple and their friends and family ("We and Us")

Exosystem (the Couple and their interactions with their own communities and cultures "We and Them")

Macrosystem (the Couple and their interactions with society/social media/media, government, culture, race, gender, society at large "We and the world")

Chronosystem (the couple and their interactions with time and pivotal events "We and Life")

The Therapist

Microsystem (The Therapist)

Mesosystem- Therapist and their friends and family

Exosystem (the Therapist and their interactions with their own communities and cultures "We and Them") and how this intersects with the couple

Macrosystem (The Therapist and their interactions with society/social media/media, government, culture, race, gender, society at large and how this intersects with the couple

Chronosystem (the therapist and their interactions with time and pivotal events and how this intersects with the couple

This display gives a visual representation of how ecological systems theory can influence the self of the therapist's work and continual professional identity. As you can see, the arrows between each set (i.e., the couple and the therapist) of systems reciprocally influence each other in the therapy room and with time through the course of treatment and the lifetime of the career of the therapist. While this chapter is focused on the questions for the therapist, the following chapters will highlight what the therapist is guided to do with the clients.

Directions: The questions below are meant as a guided reflection to delve deeper across the ecological systems and is meant for the therapist to consider with themselves. Please complete this exercise after you have reflected and written down answers from Table 2.1, noting details and keywords under each category to complete this additional exercise.

Microsystem—"We"

- What keywords do you notice about your social location and identities? What keywords or patterns do you see when you consider intersections of privilege or disadvantage?
- What keywords do you think about when you think about compromise and flexibility around identity and cultural differences? Do these keywords change when you integrate race, culture, sexuality, gender, or religion?

Mesosystem—"Us"

- What keywords do you notice about describing your current and previous friends and family influencing the work with the interracial couple/partners? How did/will you consider intersections of privilege or disadvantage?
- What generational biases (positive or negative) do I have about culture, race, sexuality, gender, and religion from growing up (related to humor, specific events, trauma, etc.) How do stories my interracial, intercultural, or interfaith clients tell me influence my relationships and my countertransference?

Exosystem—"Them"

- What keywords do you notice about your communities and your own relationship with them? How did/will you consider intersections of privilege or disadvantage with the communities you have been associated with?
- How do stories my interracial, intercultural, or interfaith clients tell me influence my history with my community and in the future?

Macrosystem—"World"

- What keywords do you notice about your relationship with government, advocacy, and social policy? How did you consider intersections of privilege or disadvantage with the entities you have been associated with?
- How do stories my interracial, intercultural, or interfaith clients tell me influence my history with the government, social policies, and advocacy?

Chronosystem—"Life"

- What keywords do you notice about your relationship with cultural humility and self-reflection? How did you consider intersections of privilege or disadvantage with the entities you have been associated with over time? How does that influence empathy and burnout?
- How do stories my interracial, intercultural, or interfaith clients tell me influence my future in the profession?

References

Aponte, H. J. (2022). The soul of therapy: The therapist's use of self in the therapeutic relationship. *Contemporary Family Therapy, 44*, 136–143. https://doi.org/10.1007/s10591-021-09614-5

Aponte, H. J., & Kissil, K. (Eds.). (2016). *The person of the therapist training model: Mastering the use of self* (1st ed.). Routledge. https://doi.org/10.4324/9781315719030

Bergkamp, J., & Ponsford, M. (2020). Cultural encapsulation. In B. J. Carducci, C. S. Nave, J. S. Mio, & R. E. Riggio (Eds.), *The Wiley encyclopedia of personality and individual differences*. John Wiley & Sons Ltd. https://doi.org/10.1002/9781119547181.ch304

Bronfenbrenner, U. (1986). Ecology of the family as a context for human development: Research perspectives. *Developmental Psychology, 22*(6), 723–742. https://doi.org/10.1037/0012-1649.22.6.723

Dansby Olufowote, R. A., Seshadri, G., & Samman, S. K. (2022). Why your interracial/multinational couples might be dropping out: A self-of-the-therapist exploration of critical factors. *Family Therapy Magazine, 21*(4). https://ftm.aamft.org/why-your-interracial-multinational-couples-might-be-dropping-out-a-self-of-the-therapist-exploration-of-critical-factors/

Demorest, A. P. (2013). The role of scripts in psychological maladjustment and psychotherapy. *Journal of Personality, 81*(6), 583–594. https://doi.org/10.1111/22924968

Franuik, R., Cohen, D., & Pomerantz, E. M. (2002). Implicit theories of relationships: Implications for relationship satisfaction and longevity. *Personal Relationships, 9*(4), 345–367. https://doi.org/10.1111/1475-6811.09401

Gutierrez, D. (2018). The role of intersectionality in marriage and family therapy multicultural supervision. *American Journal of Family Therapy, 46*(1), 14–26. https://doi.org/10.1080/01926187.2018.1437573

Hardy, K. V. (2018). The self of the therapist in epistemological context: A multicultural relational perspective. *Journal of Family Psychotherapy, 29*(1), 17–29. https://doi.org/10.1080/08975353.2018.1416211

Hays, P. A. (2001). Addressing cultural complexities in practice: A framework for clinicians and counselors. *American Psychological Association.* https://doi.org/10.1037/10411-000

Henriksen, R., Watts, R., & Bustamante, R. (2007). The multiple heritage couple questionnaire. *The Family Journal, 15*, 405–408. https://doi.org/10.1177/1066480707304794

Hsieh, A. L., & Quek, K. M. T. (2021). What we have learned: Different locations, shared experiences. In *Intersectionality in family therapy leadership* (pp. 93–103). Springer. https://doi.org/10.1007/978-3-030-67977-4_9

Jernigan, M. M., Green, C. E., Helms, J. E., Perez-Gualdron, L., & Henze, K. (2010). An examination of people of color supervision dyads: Racial identity matters as much as race. *Training and Education in Professional Psychology, 4*(1), 62–73. https://doi.org/10.1037/a0018110

Psychopathology Committee of the Group for the Advancement of Psychiatry. (2001, November). Reexamination of therapist self-disclosure. *Psychiatric Services, 52*(11):1489–1493. https://doi.org/10.1176/appi.ps.52.11.1489. PMID: 11684745

Satir, V. (1995). *Self esteem.* Celestial Arts.

Seponski, D. M., Bermudez, J. M., & Lewis, D. C. (2013). Creating culturally responsive family therapy models and research: Introducing the use of responsive evaluation as a method. *Journal of Marital and Family Therapy, 39*, 28–42. https://doi.org/10.1111/j.1752-0606.2011.00282.x

Seshadri, G., & Knudson-Martin, C. (2013). How couples manage interracial and intercultural differences: Implications for clinical practice. *Journal of Marital and Family Therapy, 39*(1), 43–58. https://doi.org/10.1111/j.1752-0606.2011.00262.x

Watts, R., & Henriksen, R. (1998). The interracial couple questionnaire. *Journal of Individual Psychology, 54*, 368–372.

Chapter 3
What Is This Attraction to Difference?

Only in positing that there is a difference between two sets of people, and that this difference has great meaning, does someone come to be interested in examining the relations between those two people.

(Yu, 2001, pp. 63–64)

Unsurprisingly, interracial, intercultural, and interfaith relationships are influenced by gender and race, which affect sexual and romantic attraction (McClintock & Sheehan, 2019; Silvestrini, 2020). Often, this phenomenon is unfairly compared to homogenous relationships in which increasing levels of similarity correlate to true love (Moses & Woesthoff, 2019). To reclaim power as interracial couples, we as therapists need to stop comparing interracial and intercultural relationships to same-race and cultural relationships; we need to honor differences as avenues of connection, rather than stressing similarity as the ideal model for loving relationships.

Attraction Versus Exoticism to Interracial Features in Macro- and Exosystems

The term exoticism is deeply rooted in colonialist ideologies based on White, patriarchal, dominant fantasy in the United States (Buggs, 2017). Sociocultural beliefs and messages stem from the macrosystem and filter through socially constructed beliefs in the mesosystem. Established at birth, the macrosystem focuses on how cultural elements affect intrapersonal development and often lasts a lifetime. Often, messages are also filtered through the mesosystem because of interactions with others. We will first address the macrosystem.

Macrosystemically, interactions are impacted by sexuality, tension, power, and rebellion from a sociocultural context. It can be difficult to meaningfully divorce these discourses or realities from interracial experiences. Specifically, women of color (WOC) in intercultural relationships have potentially been subject to conflict, domination, and cultural mediation (Ponzanesi, 2012). This parallels the oppressive historical, sociocultural dictation of values related to sexuality outside the norm. The oppression of interracial partners continues as they are expected to (for

© American Family Therapy Academy (AFTA) 2024   29
G. Seshadri, D. Gutierrez, *Interracial, Intercultural, and Interfaith Couples and Families Across the Life Cycle*, AFTA SpringerBriefs in Family Therapy,
https://doi.org/10.1007/978-3-031-58538-8_3

survival) organize their relationships by sexual stereotypes despite marital or relationship status, which influences the couples' emotional and personal wellbeing (Viveros Vigoya, 2015). Each of these reasons can be connected back to power, social context, tension, or rebellion.

In example, a therapist may be working with an interracial and intercultural couple Jessie (White, cisgender male, heterosexual) and Lola (Black, Mexican, cisgender female, heterosexual). Neither Jessie nor Lola have previously dated outside their race or culture. They have been having difficulty connecting through intimacy and sexuality. Jessie continuously tries to initiate sex with Lola; Lola feels she can't fully be present with him during these experiences and ultimately carries some guilt. Although they can communicate and share love for one another, Lola and Jessie have had difficulty discussing the context of inequity in the United States (e.g., immigration policy, attacks on Latinx communities, police brutality, and power inequity). What would these discussions have to do with intimacy? For Lola, her family, friends, and culture are and historically have been discriminated against by White communities. Jessie, with a lack of exposure and experience with communities of color, hasn't given much thought to current messages of power and discrimination. Thus, Jessie metaphorically may represent "sleeping with the oppressor," which can cause distress and anxiety to sexuality or intimacy. The therapist here must work with Jessie to understand components of Lola's anxiety, messages of power, and model empowerment for them to navigate together.

Another example related to attraction is Jorge (cisgender, Hispanic male) and Abigail (cisgender Filipino female); during the initial intake phases of treatment with each other they separately explored their interracial and intercultural attraction to each other; Jorge voiced specifically seeking out those of Asian descent due to his tendency to be attracted to "these types of females" and also because he wanted someone who was reserved, nonaggressive, and diplomatic so that he could easily communicate with them. Though Jorge was "just" explaining the "type" he was typically attracted to, one can see that his language, meaning, and discourse can be connected back to power.

Societal History and Influence

Literary records show that exoticism was conceptualized in the Enlightenment Age as colonialists entered new lands and were introduced to silk, quilts, silver, and spices that represented wealth. Yearning for wealth based on power, destinations, and people were "surveilled and supervised, patrolled and policed, regulated and restricted" and infiltrated by individuals "forging sexual links with ethnic others across ethnic borders" (Nagel, 2000, p. 113). In the nineteenth century, cinema depicted interracial and intercultural interactions as adventures steeped in fantasy and an escape from the homogeneity of whiteness. However, even with the desire for intercultural exoticism, these films shielded authentic intercultural relationships, casting actors who were White or White passing (Devos, 2015).

While exoticism may seem like an outdated concept, today's technical evolution has played an even larger part in exoticism and objectification. Chow-White (2006) explored identity discourses of race, sexuality, and gender and semantic sex tourism online. They found that Western White men use online platforms to seek racialized, sexual transgressions and appropriation of technology in domination, particularly onto Latinx, African, and Asian WOC. Interestingly, this study involved analyzing discussion boards in which hundreds of people connected through the shared cultural phenomena of power dynamics and sexuality. Thus, this issue is much larger and more entrenched than we know. These events inform cultural fetishization, objectifying communities of color, cheapening commitment, and cultivating exoticism; the attraction to, and desire for inferiority and superiority. Thinking back to Jessie and Lola, with Jessie consistently initiating sex or intimacy without a foundational understanding of Lola's experience; he may be unknowingly utilizing privilege and paralleling superiority. Although Jessie is not outright partaking in exoticist thought, his actions are perpetuating faucets of it. Similarly, Jorge exoticizing Asian traits through desirability and attraction is also noteworthy.

Reclaiming Power

Systems are not stagnant, concrete entities; oppressive historical processes can be challenged and changed. Exoticism is based on power and expectation, yet it is also nuanced, shaping sexual excitement and personal encounters. Exoticism can be a unique component of attraction, sensuality, and sexuality in intercultural relationships. Though literature and clinical training on reframing exoticism are limited, some research highlights its ability to decrease the power of oppression and increase empowerment (Forsdisk, 2001). Thus, partners and therapists working with them can shift focus from the sexist origins of exoticism to the current self-embodiment of cultural richness (Yu, 2001). In doing so, feelings of inferiority may be meditated through taking pride in intrapersonal, cultural, and relational identity. The "other" may no longer be objectified into a fantasy, but thriving in a structure of heterogeneity (Yu, 2001).

It is useful for therapists working with intercultural couples to: (1) discuss historical and present constructions of exoticism within the macrosystem; (2) deconstruct institutional messages of the exosystem; (3) challenge and move away from a cycle of Western fantasy and sexist discrimination; (4) disconnect the power and rebellious undertones; and (5) reframe narratives in order to reclaim and celebrate cultural variability and their sexuality and excitement regarding reclaimed exoticism in their relationship. Although the focus of this section was on exoticism, it is only one factor in the attraction process regarding interracial and intercultural relationships.

Subjectivity of Exchange

Wilkins et al. (2011) highlighted the meaning of traditional standards of beauty in attraction. Therapists also need to consider how beauty is standardized based on race (i.e., physical features). Exoticism suggests that features are sexualized or fetishized based on it being different than who one normally interacts with in their relationships, communities, etc. So how does this interact with theories of attraction?

For example, some attraction theories suggest that interracial attraction is based on asymmetry; inequality is exchanged based on gendered or racialized reciprocity, and symmetry—the ideal—is privileged, as it has origins in racial purity (Moses & Woesthoff, 2019). For example, the attraction to blue eyes because one has them (i.e., symmetry) and only interacts with people who have blue eyes in their communities (e.g., distance), or has exoticized them as attributing traits to having blue eyes with personality traits based on race and ethnicity (e.g., independence). In contrast, asymmetry (e.g., blue versus brown eyes) highlights discrepancy and continual indirect competition over status exchanges, especially if partners are unequal in terms of attractiveness or socioeconomic status, leaving all to assume mal intent of power in the exchange for lack of symmetry.

Lewis (2011) also highlighted the meaning of skin tone in relationship to gender from the perception of White British participants; lighter is more feminine in females and darker is more masculine in males. This is also highlighted by the concept of colorism, a product of racism that discriminates against people with darker skin tones and gives privilege to those that are lighter skinned in any society or culture, with origins from the British, the United States, and the Hindu Caste System (Shankar & Subish, 2016).

More importantly, Viveros Vigoya (2015) emphasized Peter Wades' work regarding the importance of not using exchange theory with interracial couples because the variables are difficult to quantify. He states that characteristics such as "race, age and beauty cannot fully be understood as commodities and therefore cannot be entirely 'sold' or transferred in an exchange" (as cited by Viveros Vigoya, 2015, p. S36), which also supports our suggestion to reframe exoticism. The author concluded that while interracial erotic and attraction exchanges take a linear perspective; this is a systemic process that incorporates complex factors including privacy and historical, cultural, sociological, emotional, economical, and sexual interactions.

A Note on Body Size and Interracial Attraction

In considering attraction, one must also explore the concept of body size in relationship with attraction. Glasser et al. (2009) suggested that this concept in and of itself was charged due to the intersectionality and privilege/disadvantage within the topic of body size. For example, race/body shape and physical features (e.g., skin color/tone, white-centered features), access to food/money (e.g., low vs high socioeconomic status), region (e.g., accessibility to grocery stores and/or health clubs), ableism (e.g., access to exercise), gender-based ideals and role expectations (e.g., feminine/masculine binary), age (young vs old), etc. Glasser et al. also suggested that White men had an attraction to thinner bodies as the ideal and had more negative association of larger body sizes with obesity. In addition, those that were educated perhaps would be at liberty to be more discriminating in this area because they were exchanging finances/education for beauty and attraction and for fear of being ostracized by their peers. Overall, the takeaways from Glasser et al.'s (2009) study highlight that all men in the study (i.e., White, Asian, Latino, African American) have clear body type preferences in relationship to women in heterosexual relationships; what has been more hidden that is now revealing itself is that women want more men with more masculine body types and are starting to objectify men in the ways that men have done to women.

More specifically, "race–ethnicity and gender influence body type preferences" and will show up more often with men and Whites in searching for the ideal body type (p. 30). Clinicians are encouraged to explore how these topics influence attraction, sex, and intimacy for interracial or intercultural, relationships; questions exploring and probing around what they found attractive in each other and discussions around sex and intimacy and how each other's body weight and image played a role are helpful. Further, there may be indirect or direct pressure around one partner pressuring the other partner to lose weight or look a certain way (e.g. straight hair, muscles, lightening or darkening skin). This needs to be explored as well, as it relates to racial/body size preferences (Glasser et al., 2009). Discussions around dominant ideas of beauty and its subjectivity are also helpful in externalizing and deconstructing normative ideas. Minority populations may be more accepting of larger or more shapelier body types as they have learned to negotiate with the dominant ideal of thinness.

Attraction Influences Across Multiple Systems

Viveros Vigoya (2015) captured it best when discussing attraction and intimacy in Latino interracial couples. Vigoya postulated that interracial, intercultural, and interfaith unions are plagued with mistrust and codeswitching, more specifically in the partner with a darker complexion. The assumption is that the darker person is with their lighter-skinned partner for advantage, which inevitably puts pressure on the relationship in ways that force both partners to continue to have to prove themselves in the relationship to each other and with others.

Many studies have examined the motivations for desiring interracial and intercultural unions and have related this to reasons other than love; they claim that these relationships are based on power, classism, and economic lenses. These stereotypes often are connected back to colonialism and hierarchical racial classification. For example, returning to Jorge and Abigail, we learn not only has Jorge stereotyped his attraction to Abigail with assumptions about her race (reserved, nonaggressive, and diplomatic) but also that Abigail participates in this stereotyped by saying that she was attracted to his dark skin tone, body, and muscles because it represented feeling protected; she likened it to a knight in shining armor, which played into him being a member of the armed forces. Within these perceptions, interracial attraction is viewed as abnormal and atypical. An invisible boundary of difference is thus continually negotiated and discussed by the couple, implicitly or explicitly (Yu, 2001).

In sum, we are asking both the reader and mental health professionals to consider the stereotypes and meaning behind how interracial and intercultural partners, couples, and families communicate their attraction directly and indirectly in their relationships with each other, community, and society. Thinking back to Jessie and Lola, Lola had been experiencing distress and anxiety regarding being with a White man. Therapists can deconstruct commercialized messages from their systems relationships that the partners may have internalized or developed. For example, questions surrounding relationship and identity development can involve constructing a family timeline. "Throughout your family history, has anyone dated outside their race? If so (or if not), what messages did family members share about dating outside race? Were messages explicitly communicated or was it a known rule not talked about? What has Whiteness or diversity meant or represented to you and your family? Are there messages you want to move away from or desire to keep as you continue your relationship with Jessie?"

Commercialization

Popular films often depict individuals involved in interracial relationships as deviants with sexualized animalistic attractions that create their interest in people outside their own race. We believe this can influence people's perceptions around attraction. Unfortunately, past and present discourses reinforce the predominant oppression and pathology related to these relationships. There may be aspects of privilege to also be explored here. For example, Sally (Hispanic, cisgender, female) had to go through her own process of not only coming out and being in a lesbian relationship with Laura (White, cisgender, female) but also not being with someone of Hispanic background. While Laura may have also had to go through similar processes (i.e., coming out, being a lesbian, and not being with someone of a White background), Laura is also privileged in that, overall, there is more racial and cultural acceptance from her racial group for her coming out as a lesbian, than there is for Sally. For Sally, coming out includes the macro influence of being a WOC, woman of color, and navigating the coming out process and as a result may face lack of cultural group acceptance for these exact reasons.

We use these examples to help the reader acknowledge that if partners share these experiences as a part of their background to not view this in a negative lens, but rather explore how these larger systems dynamics may affect the relationship in addition to intersectionality; for example, Joe (cisgender African American, male) may have specifically sought out Katarina (cisgender, Greek, female) despite feeling that there weren't any prospects for himself within his own race/culture, but later discovers that choosing Katarina connects to wanting to make sense of previous generational racial traumas that relate back to slavery. This translates to him feeling like he is walking on eggshells where he is afraid that she will leave him at any moment, not only due to him being the minority partner but also due to her wanting only a green card. Intersectionality wise, although she is of privileged background (i.e., White racial background), she also responds by withdrawing, as she feels helpless because she is in a foreign land (i.e., not a citizen) and a woman in a patriarchy-based country. This reinforces his position to not feel good enough, because of her perceived rejections, especially around race, which is what is making him more avoidant.

There are many reasons individuals choose interracial and intercultural partners. This speaks volumes in how this can influence an interracial/intercultural/interfaith couple and their family within their microsystem (i.e., within their relationships), exosystem (i.e., communities), and macrosystem (e.g., laws/social media), as exemplified in the example of Joe and Katarina.

Continuing to use Joe and Katarina, Joe's generational racial trauma translated to being avoidant in his family of origin and letting his sisters and other females in authority take over; Katarina does not know what to do with this, as she grew up in a patriarchy-based home where her father was dominant, making all the decisions for the family, and she had faded into the background, especially in her adolescent years. As a young adult, she chose Joe because she was hoping to express more independence. The therapist would use this as an avenue for exploring how these macrosystem themes show up in the relationship presently.

Identity Discourses on Attraction

Attraction further revolves around identity discourse. Seshadri and Knudson-Martin (2013) noted that many couples they studied discussed racial differences as an attraction, which was also a strength-based relational strategy for managing differences. Several participants wanted to choose a partner who wasn't like their parents; they believed that other races would not have specific parental traits they didn't like. They also generalized these traits to their larger racial or ethnic group, as they had also experienced these traits in individuals who were from their background.

Silvestrini (2020) and Brooks and Neville (2017) did studies that highlighted the role that race and racial stereotypes can have in sexual or romantic attraction and found a link between them, highlighting that race implicitly influences attraction (Seshadri & Samman, 2021).

It is the job of mental health professionals to probe for these macrosystem factors, highlight them, and link them to the processes between who is in the room. If they are negatively impacting the couple, it often connects back to stereotypes. Does this mean the clinician must ask "What stereotypes do you believe in?" No. Process and circular questions based on curiosity will help make beliefs explicit to both the therapist and partner(s). For example, "Tell me about some expectations in your family? Were there certain ways you were expected to behave, act, or communicate? Are/were there shoulds regarding body shape, weight, and size? What or who has/have impacted expectations throughout your lifetime, your relationships romantic or through friendship?" Exploring expectations, awareness, and acknowledgment of perceived expectations connected to culture can shed light on potential implicit stereotypes.

For example, research with African Americans discovered that the darker the skin color, the greater the association of skin color and racial identity to negative associations—lower SES, education, etc. These ideas complicate attraction and mate selection among African American females, and often portray available mates negatively.

Lehmiller et al. (2014) also examined the impact of peer group evaluation and the sociopolitical context of world events on attraction in Black-White couples. Positive or negative beliefs about race relations were overridden by current peer evaluations, suggesting the importance of others' perceptions of the partners. Lastly, it is important to explore how others perceive the relationship in that it may play into issues of approval, which continues to be a strong theme of oppression for interracial and intercultural couples.

Clinical Implications

It is important for therapists to recognize, and explore with couples and families: (1) discourse and how race and culture are mutually constructed and play off of each other; (2) how social norms dictate what is attractive and sexually desirable (including body shape and size), and the impact of these norms on client(s); (3) beliefs and expectations (implicit and explicit) communicated in the initial phases of dating or the relationship/marriage, or currently communicated; (4) how "others" (e.g., friends, family, peers, community, society) influence relationship choices based on their support or lack of support for the relationship, or based on discrimination (Seshadri & Knudson-Martin, 2013); (5) how negative and positive biases of clients, therapists, and "others" abound, based on visual racial differences, evaluator affiliations, and stereotypes; and (6) discourses on attraction and how this influences family roles and interactions with "others."

Utilizing Stories Within Social Constructionism

A social constructionist narrative lens maintains that humans have stories that are saturated with values, experiences, and authenticity that shape identities interwoven within dominant narratives. For example, earlier in this chapter, Abigail's story of attraction stemmed from wanting to be protected. In treatment, it would take time to realize the impact of her own voice.

The macrosystem—systemic and cultural traditions—refers to creating a framework for making meaning of our individual lives; it reflects what "should" happen in life and how to successfully coordinate our actions with others. Some examples of macrosystemic values are heterosexual relationships, traditional gender roles, procreation, strict intergenerational patterns, etc. Culture provides a set of values intercultural couples can use to interpret their lives and know whether they are living a "good" life (Sue et al., 2019). For Katarina, culture and family of origin frame patriarchy and masculinity as central. Through exploring these stories, therapists can focus on dominant discourses interwoven in larger systems and cultures, giving perspective to the contexts that contribute to attraction. Interpretation of attraction expectation may lead systems to be naturally oppressive and correlated with their ability to be flexible. Specifically, therapists can explore problematic, rigid intrapersonal and interpersonal beliefs partners maintain about each other's culture (Tong, 2019). By externalizing conversations and separating the problem from the person, we can deconstruct beliefs about color of our skin, racial identities, and intergenerational messages on attraction.

The deconstruction process enables therapists and couples to confront oppressive dominant discourses and re-envision attraction. For example, therapists can utilize expectation questions once again to explore this process in various experiences. Therapists can ask, "When in the presence of each other's family members, are there expectations on how you greet or interact with grandparents, parents, siblings, etc.? Has tension or distress occurred when these expectations weren't met by one another? If they were, were they acknowledged or celebrated?" By exploring these expectations, the therapist and partner(s) can recognize the value given to them, what they feel should happen, and the level of value they feel their partner is giving to them and their beliefs. Further, they can externalize and reframe these values and expectations so that specific cultural beliefs can be centered, deconstructed, and reauthored by the partners.

For example, therapists can explore problematic, rigid intrapersonal and interpersonal beliefs partners maintain about each other's culture (Tong, 2019). For example, asking questions detailed in Appendix 3.1 around how the couple became attracted to each other, if others had opinions about the attraction, what did they think about each other when they met, what made them decide to pursue a relationship, etc. This process enables therapists and couples to confront oppressive dominant discourses and re-envision attraction.

Case Application

In clinical practice, client preferences abound about not having a partner with a desired "hair type" or seeking a specific ethnic or racial background with assumed characteristics such as independence or submissiveness as themes in both couples and individual therapy. These preferences often stem from one's family of origin or a desire for a certain level of acculturation or a desired experience related to healing one's own wounds. Exploring these discourses and the familial and societal messages about what is attractive has been very revealing. These messages often come from the majority culture and media.

Robert (a cisgender, dark-skinned Native American male) said he was attracted to Asian women and one of the reasons he chose his (cisgender, light-skinned, Japanese) wife, Linda, because he believed she would be submissive. Through the years, he acknowledged it was very difficult for him to accept her desire to be a singer, as he felt he couldn't protect her from some of the career issues. She would be on the road a lot, appear in potentially seedy areas around strangers, and needed to demonstrate her sex appeal as part of the job. He also said it was important to him to have a spouse who stayed home to take care of the kids—a view he ascribed to his cultural experiences and family of origin.

Initially, it was difficult for you to hear him talk about seeking submissive women to control them and be in control, or even the need to be needed, which he couched as a protective stance. You felt anxious about the potential challenges this issue posed. Being a minority female in the therapist role made you wonder about the assumptions he was bringing to the therapeutic process. Realizing this, you explored his family of origin and any messages he received about women, particularly minority women, and how his identity as a Hispanic male, family of origin, and culture contributed to these aspects. You also examined the messages about the singing profession he received from friends and witnessed in bars, as well as messages about his wife's sexuality. He acknowledged the role of his male dominance and how that came across in his perspective toward his wife.

Through this process, you and he discovered he didn't have any problem with his wife singing in general and that he trusted her and did not want to control her. According to him, they both came to an agreement where she would be the lead singer in church, a place they both valued, where she could express her individuality, and share her passion of singing with others, worship, and the word of God, while still having time for him and their children. What also seemed to be a power struggle resolved with discussions around why he felt he needed to protect her and how this came across as stifling her individuality; this seemed to connect to the presence of alcohol/substances at the seedy bars. With your suggestion, he also seemed able to reframe individuality by connecting it to their spirituality—a value that they both believed in from their religious doctrine. The other concerns disappeared as he wanted to support his spouse's voice without orchestrating her. Though you were not seeing his spouse in therapy, you were grateful that she could express her voice, and that he was able to hear it, and challenge and revise some of his assumptions around his initial attraction.

Lessons from the Chapter

In this chapter, we discussed attraction, exoticism, and the systemic influences involved in attraction (i.e., status exchange, commercialization, sexual exoticism). Stereotypes, biases, negative discourses, and assumptions around similarity. As clinicians, exoticism must be challenged and connected back to the way that the couple relates to each other and supports reframed ways of thinking. In deconstructing negative stories around preferences, interracial and intercultural partners can feel freer to express their attractions within multiple avenues of their relationship, community, culture, and society. Extended exercises are included in Appendix 3.1.

Appendix 3.1: Attraction and Your Interracial/Intercultural/ Interfaith Clients

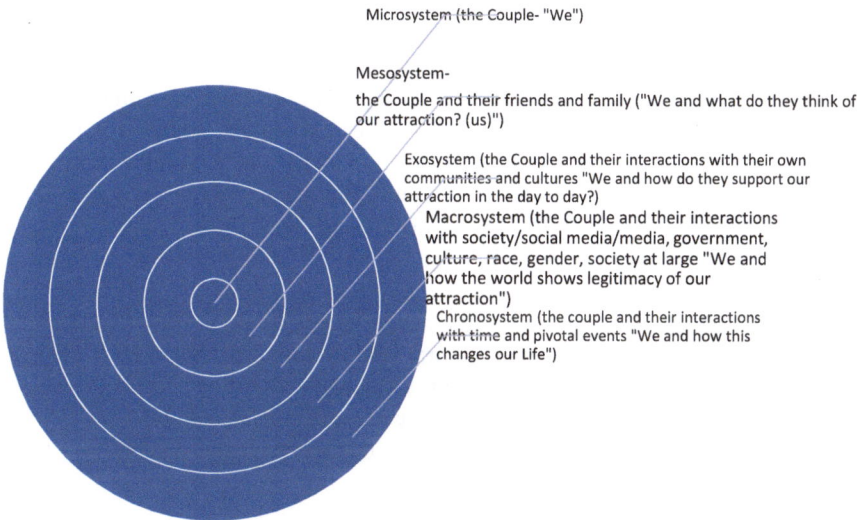

Microsystem (the Couple- "We")

Mesosystem-
the Couple and their friends and family ("We and what do they think of our attraction? (us)")

Exosystem (the Couple and their interactions with their own communities and cultures "We and how do they support our attraction in the day to day?)

Macrosystem (the Couple and their interactions with society/social media/media, government, culture, race, gender, society at large "We and how the world shows legitimacy of our attraction")

Chronosystem (the couple and their interactions with time and pivotal events "We and how this changes our Life")

The questions below provide a guided reflection across the ecological systems to inform your interventions with interracial and intercultural partners around the topic of attraction. Please complete this exercise after you have reflected and written down answers from Table 2.1. As you respond to the questions, please consider keywords from Table 2.1. For further exercise, imagine the graphic on this page, as a replacement of the top graphic in Appendix 2.1.

Microsystem—"We"

- What keywords do you notice about the couple's social location and identities in their discussions of attraction to each other? What intersections of privilege or disadvantage for them?
- Are their attraction stories related to colorism, stereotypes, exoticism, and bias? How do these relate to race, culture, sexuality, gender, or religion?

Mesosystem—"Us"

- What generational biases (positive or negative) do they have about culture, race, sexuality, gender, and religion from growing up (related to humor, specific events, trauma, etc.)
- What stories, stereotypes, and/or biases do you notice the couple discussing when considering attraction and their current or previous friends and family influence? How did/will you consider intersections of privilege or disadvantage? How do these stories influence the relationship between themselves, their peers, and family members?

Exosystem—"Them"

- What stories, stereotypes, and/or biases do you notice the couple discussing when considering attraction and their community influence? How did/will you consider intersections of privilege or disadvantage?
- What community messages (positive or negative) do interracial, intercultural, and interfaith partners have about culture, race, sexuality, gender, and religion from growing up in their communities, previously and currently (related to humor, specific events, acculturation, trauma, etc.)? How do these stories influence their relationship to the communities?

Macrosystem—"World"

- What stories, stereotypes, and/or biases with government, advocacy, and social policy influence interracial, intercultural, and interfaith partners? How did you consider intersections of privilege or disadvantage with the entities (with societal or cultural guidelines and beliefs) they have been associated with?
- How do current laws and policies influence the stories of your clients?

Chronosystem—"Life"

- What stories and phrases do you notice about the interracial, intercultural, and interfaith partners over the timeline of their relationship? How do they address bias, stereotypes, and other macro messages about their relationship? With others?
- How did/will you consider intersections of privilege or disadvantage within their timeline?

References

Brooks, J. E., & Neville, H. A. (2017). Interracial attraction among college men: The influence of ideologies, familiarity, and similarity. *Journal of Social and Personal Relationships, 34*(2), 166–183. https://doi.org/10.1177/0265407515627508

Buggs, S. G. (2017). Does (mixed) race matter? The role of race in interracial sex, dating, and marriage. *Sociology Compass, 11*(11), e12531. https://doi.org/10.1111/soc4.12531

Chow-White, P. A. (2006). Race, gender, and sex on the net: Semantic networks of selling and storytelling sex tourism. *Media, Culture & Society, 28*(6), 883–905. https://doi.org/10.1177/0163443706068922

DeVos, A. D. (2015). *Mixed messages: An interdisciplinary narrative of interracial sexuality in US films, 1956–2001* (Publication No. 3741481) [Doctoral dissertation, University of Maryland]. ProQuest Dissertations and Theses Global.

Forsdisk, C. (2001). Travelling concepts: Postcolonial approaches to exoticism. *Paragraph, 24*(3), 12–29.

Glasser, C. L., Robnett, B., & Feliciano, C. (2009). Internet daters' body type preferences: Race–ethnic and gender differences. *Sex Roles, 61*(1–2), 14–33. https://doi.org/10.1007/s11199-009-9604-x

Lehmiller, J., Graziano, W., & VanderDrift, L. (2014). Peer influence and attraction to interracial romantic relationships. *Social Sciences, 3*(1), 115–127. https://doi.org/10.3390/socsci3010115

Lewis, M. B. (2011). Who is the fairest of them all? Race, attractiveness, and skin color sexual dimorphism. *Personality & Individual Differences, 50*(2), 159–162. https://doi.org/10.1016/j.paid.2010.09.018

McClintock, E. A., & Sheehan, S. Z. (2019). Race, gender, and social exchange in young adult unions. *Sociological Spectrum, 39*(2), 71–92. https://doi.org/10.1080/02732173.2019.1608340

Moses, J., & Woesthoff, J. (2019). Romantic relationships across boundaries: Global and comparative perspectives. *The History of the Family, 24*(3), 439–465. https://doi.org/10.1080/1081602X.2019.1634120

Nagel, J. (2000). Ethnicity and sexuality. *Annual Review of Sociology, 26*(1), 107–133.

Ponzanesi, S. (2012). The color of love: Madamismo and interracial relationships in the Italian colonies. *Research in African Literatures, 43*(2), 155–172. https://doi.org/10.2979/reseafrilite.43.2.155

Seshadri, G., & Knudson-Martin, C. (2013). How couples manage interracial and intercultural differences: Implications for clinical practice. *Journal of Marital and Family Therapy, 39*, 43–58. https://doi.org/10.1111/j.1752-0606.2011.00262.x

Seshadri, G., & Samman, S. (2021, March). *I don't have to marry my parent: Multi-racial attraction-based coupling* [Workshop]. International Family Therapy Association, Virtual.

Shankar, P. R., & Subish, P. (2016). Fair skin in South Asia: An obsession? *Journal of Pakistan Association of Dermatology, 17*(2), 100–104.

Silvestrini, M. (2020). "It's not something I can shake": The effect of racial stereotypes, beauty standards, and sexual racism on interracial attraction. *Sexuality & Culture, 24*(1), 305–325. https://doi.org/10.1007/s12119-019-09644-0

Sue, D. W., Sue, D., Neville, H. A., & Smith, L. (2019). *Counseling the culturally diverse: Theory and practice* (8th ed.). Wiley.

Tong, H. P. (2019). *The Gottman method, narrative therapy, and psychodynamic approach in counseling interracial couples* (Publication No. 119) [Master's thesis, Winona State University]. Counselor Education Capstones.

Viveros Vigoya, M. (2015). The sexual erotic market as an analytical framework for understanding erotic-affective exchanges in interracial sexually intimate and affective relationships. *Culture, Health & Sexuality, S1*, 34–46. https://doi.org/10.1080/13691058.2014.979882

Wilkins, C. L., Chan, J. F., & Kaiser, C. R. (2011). Racial stereotypes and interracial attraction: Phenotypic prototypicality and perceived attractiveness of Asians. *Cultural Diversity & Ethnic Minority Psychology, 17*(4), 427–431. https://doi.org/10.1037/a0024733

Yu, H. (2001). *Thinking Orientals: Migration, contact, and exoticism in modern America*. Oxford University Press.

Chapter 4
Interracial and Intercultural Dating and Couple Formation: How Can We Negotiate Our Differences?

How would your parents react to your dating a Black guy? Oh, they'd give me the third degree. At least I know my dad would because he thinks that if you're too different you can't work it out.

[Denise, a Latina woman] (Morales, 2012, p. 320)

Historical Attitudes Toward Dating

Before Richard and Mildred Loving took their love to court in 1967 and won the right to marry—thus granting marriage rights between races across the nation—they met, dated, and fell in love. In fact, Richard and Mildred were neighborhood sweethearts and knew one another through their families (Gilmer, 2017), a characteristic that is extremely prevalent in the beginning of many romantic relationship narratives. They found love at a time when they could be beaten, arrested, or killed for their relationship, yet they stayed strong, navigated their identities together, and remained married until Richard's death in 1975. For over 300 years in the US culture, colonial and state legislatures prohibited any form of dating, sexual interaction, or marriage between White and ethnically and racially diverse people (Gilmer, 2017). Thus, as interracial relationships begin to form, an entire history of inequities and oppression is already embedded within their story.

Discrimination was systemically based on racial segregation and slavery, ultimately to maintain White superiority and purity, conservative religious value, and power. Historically, public laws and overall systemic structures heavily impacted and created barriers to interracial/intercultural dating in the United States. For example, Alabama laws regarding illegal interracial marriage were still written in legal books and were not removed until the year 2000 (Alabama Secretary of State, n.d.). This is alarming since this is as recent as 24 years ago. Despite laws promoting social interaction amongst the races (e.g., anti-miscegenation laws in 1964), many still indirectly or directly experience social disapproval for their interracial relationship. Furthermore, worldwide and through the ages, similar reasons preventing interracial and intercultural marriage included: a desire to maintain racial and ethnic purity, implications with property, limits with geographic location, and

© American Family Therapy Academy (AFTA) 2024

G. Seshadri, D. Gutierrez, *Interracial, Intercultural, and Interfaith Couples and Families Across the Life Cycle*, AFTA SpringerBriefs in Family Therapy, https://doi.org/10.1007/978-3-031-58538-8_4

socially constructed implications for maintaining cultural homogeneity, and others' perceived difficulties around cultural adaptation.

Religion has also created barriers for interracial, intercultural, and interfaith dating, relationships, and marriage. Simpson and Yinger (2013) detailed the speech of the presiding judge for the Loving case that basically suggested that God intended for the races to be separated by distance, so they *should not* intermix. Further, there are some religions that still speak of being unequally yoked with relationship partners as a deterrent (Riley, 2013).

The Influence of Movies and Social Media

Exosystemically, interracial/intercultural dating is thought of as Black and White coupling versus multiple cultural identities. As a society based on binaries, having opposite skin color is visible and you can clearly see and understand where power lies (Jordan, 2019). Buggs (2017), further discussed historical assumptions of sex and race intersection, particularly around colonialism, as White men's accessibility to Women of Color bodies and racial fetishization. Although embedded in history, theoretical structures of White dominance and social approval continue today through media and dating preferences (Allen & Uskul, 2019). As media exposure has increased, so have stereotypes of interracial dating and cultures. For example, movies such as *Save the Last Dance*, *Guess Who is Coming to Dinner/Guess Who* (i.e., the remake), *Jungle Fever*, and *The Bodyguard* are wellknown and have impacted societal perception of mixed-race couples, mainly White and Black coupling, dating, and attraction. In addition, these films emphasize and depict racial stigmatization as centering within their relationships, excluding components of relationship development, identity, and evolvement.

These films have impacted generations in the dating, attraction, and formation stages of relationship. Thus, clients are coming in with histories of societal and structural discrimination embedded in how their intercultural attraction has been developed and shaped. Clients will potentially need to reform and reevaluate what different sources have taught them (e.g., movies, newspapers, social media). Today, films that depict other racial combinations where the interracial/intercultural relationship is the center of the story include newer movies, such as *Mississippi Masala*, *Fools Rush In*, *My Big Fat Greek Wedding* (1, 2) and *Our Family Wedding*. It's important to ask clients how they feel about their interracial, intercultural, or interfaith combination and related nuances which inevitably unearths messaging and stereotypes within dating and the other's racial, cultural, and religious differences.

In relation to media, online dating such as apps like Match, Bumble, Hinge, HER, etc. have contributed to lack of interracial connection and what constitutes attractiveness. A simple swipe and setting of filters can put people in their ideal pool of romantic relationship candidates; much of which continues to center Whiteness, bias, and power. In addition, other sites such as eHarmony and Hinge, have rebranded to now include interracial dating or certain race or ethnicity filters regarding race (Zhou, 2022), though at one point some sites, including these, would *warn* members to not avoid choosing specific races when setting preferences, including the avoidance or request of those of their own background, couching this as *limiting matches*. Unfortunately, this reinforces bias and power, unbeknownst to users who participate in this emotional dance. Clinicians need to ask their clients questions around racial preferences and choice, probing for colorism, as well as other assumptions and biases, and suggestions from others that choosing a White partner was for social and/or racial acceptance (if applicable).

Disparities in perceptions of attraction are even found in sexually expansive communities. For example, one study of 331 gay male Tinder users found that White looking users were still considered most appealing to date (Ranzini & Rosenbaum, 2020). In addition, a study by Wu et al. (2015) found that racially diverse individuals saw White potential romantic partners as highly attractive and desirable and were unphased by dating outside their own race. However, with a new generation of youth, media and teen-centered shows are beginning to portray various interracial couplings, giving evidence to a shift to interracial relationships perception and navigation for young adults beginning to navigate romantic relationships.

There are also POC, particularly WOC (e.g., Latina/e, Asian, Black, etc. women), who don't necessarily want to interracially date but feel stuck with the amount of available dating partners within their racial, ethnic, and cultural backgrounds. Some relate this to education levels (i.e., wanting to marry someone at or above their education level) and levels of their professions/status (e.g., after working so hard to become a lawyer (white collar), I don't want to marry someone who has a blue-collar job). Others choose not to interracially date due to not wanting to bridge racial, ethnic, and cultural gaps, or even feel rejected by White men (Boyd et al., 2021; Muro & Martinez, 2016). These reasons could propel them to search for dating, relationship, or marriage partners within their own backgrounds or end up staying single, further perpetuating stereotypes of their own backgrounds. Clinically, the therapist must probe for these attitudes, as they can be influenced by historical segregation, lack of access, and opportunities to education. Sometimes this may translate into a subtle rejection or fear of rejection of the interracial partner which can play out in dating dynamics.

For example, Sarita (cisgender, South Asian female) was dating Hubert (cisgender, Hawaiian male) and had been deeply in love with him for a couple of years. Upon meeting her family, Hubert was rejected by them due to his lack of desire to continue his education further. He had already obtained his master's degree but would not pursue a doctorate or a post doc. Since education was a high value of Sarita's family, they were trying to convince her to break up with him and they would arrange a marriage for her with a South Asian male who would have a doctorate degree and was doing a post doc. Sarita was in quite a conundrum. Should she risk family disapproval and ostracization for community support, cultural connection, and acceptance? Discussions around boundaries with Sarita's family, her pleasing voice, connection to her culture, and exploring the factors influencing whether she was willing to let go of her relationship with Hubert or not, centered on treatment considerations.

Familial, Community, and Cultural Instructions

Macrosystemically, these societal influences impact a dating couple in several ways. One is the messages and meaning that they bring to their relationships and must continually negotiate their own identities while negotiating their relationships. Sometimes this also includes having to deal with mesosystemically and exosystemically feeling excluded from cultural and family expectation. We saw this with Sarita. Also, projection of negative stereotypes while dating, and even throughout the relationship, makes people feel like they must monitor what they communicate through action and words (Buggs, 2017; McGrath et al., 2016). Even the act of "going outside the culture" has social pressure and implications that may lead to feelings of shame, the need to conceal the relationship, or fear loss of their own relationship with their culture, or even competition with others (Boyd et al., 2021; Gonlin, 2023; Mayer & Viviers, 2017). Many believe the negative, that an interracial partner is chosen for deviance or insurrection from one's own background. Clinicians will serve clients well to probe for the reasoning and implications behind choosing to date an interracial, intercultural, and/or interfaith partner, while being cautious to avoid their own potential negative stereotypes and beliefs.

We can look at Denise, the Latina woman quoted, who shared her family's thoughts on dating a Black man. She shared that her dad would think he (a Black man) would be too different. Already, there is a set expectation that cultural differences would arise within their relationship and within Denise's family perception of their relationship; and this is only to one specific racial background. Systemically thinking, Denise would have to navigate her feelings and actions within her relationship and maintain awareness of how those feelings and actions might change in front of her family with her partner. Further, Denise specifically mentioned her father would have difficulty. Thus, messages on cultural masculinity and power may also impact partner and familial relationship navigation.

To survive this, the couple must attempt to become insular from negative influences. Not surprisingly, the dating phase in interracial/intercultural/interethnic relationships involves discovering how to circularly shield the relationship from covert and overt attacks from others (Foeman & Nance, 2002). During the dating phase of a relationship, there are multiple points for identity development, both as a couple and in how the couple wants to present themselves to others. This identity development process is multifaceted across varying social locations. For minority partners, acknowledging the intersections of race and gender are also important during this negotiation process (Chuang et al., 2021).

Lots of times couples experience pressure in even being open about problems within the relationship. One couple described the theme of societal pressure, saying that when they mentioned their problems or issues to other people, others would automatically assume that the problem was one of culture or race as a way of stereotyping. Often, regardless of the interracial combination, couples experience looks, stares, attitudes, perceptions, the nonverbal, and body language. Despite the reduction of direct experiences of discrimination, this suggests that experiences of prejudice and discrimination still occur.

Harris and Kalbfleisch (2000) studied Black-White participants, and many cited familial disapprovals beyond not being attracted when choosing to avoid an interracial relationship. More specifically, they feared being cut off or estranged from family, problems in career advancement due to discrimination, fears regarding friends/community disapproval, and negative reactions from strangers when in the local community/the public. To avoid this ostracization, some decide not to engage in interracial coupling. Sadly, they may have to choose between dating their partner and their families of origin.

Microsystem and Mesosystem: Family Importance and Intergenerational Differences

Social approval involves being within societal "norms" and is connected to family cultural values. This may impact interracial/intercultural dating, yet even more prominent is approval of family of origin. More recently, parental approval may or may not hold significance. A study by Field et al. (2013) found that perceived parental approval of interracial relationships differed with respect to sex/gender (more males reported being favorable) and race (White students were least favorable) among participants from historically Black colleges, which historically connects back to relations from slavery, where sexual relations between Whites and Blacks was considered only *acceptable* in the context of rape. However, for individuals already within a relationship outside of dominant structures (i.e., Whiteness and heterosexuality), parental approval may not be as impactful. Clinicians need to explore how this would impact partners and their families.

In contrast, a study by Rosenfeld and Kim (2005) found that individuals in interracial or same-sex couples placed significantly less value on parental approval of their partners and shifted away from passing this value along to their children. However, with cultural families, the family nucleus may be comprised of more than parents but also siblings, grandparents, aunts, uncles, cousins, and so on. Research has shown that extended families not only provide social support but contribute significantly to family members' cultural identity development, emotional connection, and unique opportunities of bonding through intergenerational patterns. Clinicians need to also consider this in the context of the coming out process as well with same-sex partners.

Family and families of choice play an integral role in familial and individual emotional stability (James et al., 2018). Couples may face negotiation of boundaries including potential lack of visibility and invalidation, intrusion, and disrespect with multiple members (Addison & Coolhart, 2009). For example, a Latina lesbian who identifies as nonbinary and masculine presenting in an intercultural relationship with a Black feminine ciswoman may experience acceptance in sexual identity but faces intrusion on her gender expression and role of "breadwinner" within her relationship versus being traditionally provided for as seen in larger Latinx society (Morales, 2012).

Studies have further found correlations between disconnection from family and culture or lack of positive family relationships, and adverse mental health outcomes (Guo et al., 2015; Stein et al., 2015). Thus, there are various members and key figures in individuals' lives that interracial/intercultural relationships would have to navigate. It would be advantageous for clinicians to probe for disruptions in mental health related to family conflict, discrimination, or community conflict in relationship to the clients' interracial, intercultural, and/or interfaith partners.

Connecting back to the exosystemic (i.e., community), macrosystemic (i.e., ideology), and influence of religion, Perry (2014) found that a desire for homogeneity with religion influenced White people around their openness to date interracially. Perry was unsure if diverse congregations played a role in the decision-making of choice of an interracial/interethnic dating partner or other factors. Clinicians need to ask interracial, intercultural, and interfaith clients how they are planning to interact with others (i.e., parents, neighbors, community, society) and what their plan of action/support would be.

Microsystem and Macrosystem: Multiple Relational Identity Negotiations

For couples who identify as multidiverse within their own identities and within their relationships, additional layers are added and navigated (Csizmadia et al., 2015). Within their relationships, they need to navigate their dimensions of differences, including discussions on privilege through culture, beliefs, and expectations of coming out, and prioritization of relationship over family rituals (Addison & Coolhart, 2009). Societally, historically, and culturally, there are layers of discriminatory structures in place that contribute to individual and relational identity negotiation while dating. For example, the LGBTQ community has faced prejudice and minority stressors regarding sexual and gender identities, yet exclusion of intersectionality experiences is constant (Cyrus, 2017). BIPOC LGBTQ communities face structural barriers and rights for LGBTQ communities still center around Whiteness and continue to exclude race, despite the intersection in many individuals (Prasad, 2018). They may keep the relationship to themselves or test to see if others are accepting before revealing interracial relationship status, including when meeting friends and parents (Foeman & Nance, 2002). Thinking back to the Foeman and Nance (2002) stages, the first stage of "coming out" to family includes coming out as an interracial/intercultural partnership but could involve another layer of sexuality and gender.

BIPOC LGBTQ partners face multiple 'isms, including sexism, racism, and heterosexism including minority stressors, coming out to family, sexuality and gender role exploration, and renegotiation and exploration of sex-passion-intimacy and love (Burke, 2015; Csizmadia et al., 2015; Hertlein et al., 2020). Further research highlighted intersectional experiences for dating through created expectation of rejection per identity; implicit or explicit messages; concealment of identity within relationship and to others; societal negative attitudes; acculturative stress and migration; separate and foundational cultural ideologies; intersectional trauma; and potential family alienation (Gutierrez et al., 2022; Lundquist & Lin, 2015). Regarding power inequities, couples who are White and ethically coupled face negotiation through centered Whiteness in race, sexuality, and potentially gender identity expression (i.e., one partner holding privilege identifying as cisgender).

Overall, as a couple, recognition of being romantically involved is another space for negotiation. Even as small as a waitress asking "if the check is going to be together or split" can feel like multiple microaggressions and contribute to exclusion or invisibility. Then comes the internal and external discussion of "is it worth it to clarify?" which is concluded via the amount of energy, emotional exhaustion, and safety. Another question for the clinician to probe is if either partner is willing to support the emotions resulting from this experience. Steinbugler (2005) interviewed same-sex and heterosexual interracial couples' experiences of visibility; her participants highlighted the need for attunement to the social demographic of diversity within neighborhoods, queer spaces, and the overall social makeup of communities. Her work further gives voice to the negotiation of sexual, racial, and gender differences. Even a recent study by Robinson (2015), of gay men's preferences in online dating, found that White coupling was desired potentially to avoid negotiating racial differences, cultural assumptions and stereotypes, and limited exposure to mixed-race coupling. Additionally, all of this was being done through a filter and search preferences. Clinicians need to ask and probe for assumptions around White culture (e.g., do they believe they don't have a culture?) as well as for minority partners (i.e., stereotypes).

Lastly, potential relational ambiguity (Addison & Coolhart, 2009), where behaviors and actions aren't mutually defined but based on cultural expectations rather than relational prioritization may contribute to negotiations. Strong familial and personal identities within Latino culture, for example, include religious and gender identities. For instance, religiosity can create oppressive stances within a family, yet it can also be a source of support creating life meaning, family, community, and tradition for POCs. When partners differ in religious value, there may be tension in the relationship due to identity processes that contributed to family, development, and culture. Potential differences in lack of religious prioritization among interracial couples may impact individual and relational well-being and further promote stress (Henderson & Brantley, 2019). Thus, relational negotiations are vast and not encapsulated within race, but various differences in cultures coming together in relationship.

Exploring Social Construction with the Lens of Fairness/Equity

How do we integrate fairness, equity, and balance in application to interracial couples—especially where there are nonquantifiable intersections of identity? Or intersections of privilege and oppression within both partners? Are we using fairness based on heteronormativity and privilege? What if there are generational ledgers that need to be balanced that show up while dating that stem from either historical oppression or generational trauma?

Application of ecological systems theory means exploring relational justice at each level; microsystemically within the couple, mesosytemically with family and friends around stereotypes and expectations, exosystemically with community and being in public when there are stares or reactions to the couple, and macrosystemically based on bias, societal discourse that they have internalized from larger society during the dating process. This continual *relational reflection* process can help with deciding how to deal with discrimination, isolation, boundaries, and when to use humor or avoidance. For extended practice and suggested exercises, please refer to Appendix 4.1.

Case Application

It is not a common occurrence in therapy for you to see a couple who are dating and not already on the way to getting engaged or close to the altar and have not had the experience of cohabitation. However, Manny, a 30-year-old cisgender, able-bodied, Buddhist Chinese male, is dating Adeline, a 29-year-old Filipina, cisgender, Catholic, female with chronic illness. They came to see you due to tensions in their relationship. They cited historically tense relations between the Chinese and Filipinos, which was carried into their relationship. When Manny's father lived in China, he had a Filipino servant whom he was swindled by, which created fears and stereotypes around Filipino people. He is unaware of Manny's relationship with Adeline; but Manny knows of the incident with the servant and is hesitant to introduce Adeline due to his father's perceptions, stereotypes, and microaggressive comments about Filipino people. Adeline loves to do things that please Manny, which include cooking, cleaning, etc., when she comes over to his apartment. Her friends think he is taking advantage of her, especially when she misses time with them to take care of Manny or has a flare-up with her chronic illness. You can relate as you have managed chronic illness too and understand the difficulties. Adeline really wants to meet Manny's father and feels hurt that Manny won't introduce her, as she feels that this would demonstrate his commitment to her.

For you it was difficult to not see the power issues and the generational ledger of the father subtly expecting Manny to balance the ledger between the father (mesosystem), Filipino and Chinese relations (macrosystem and exosystem), and the servant (mesosystem). Manny seems to have been internalizing destructive entitlement by expecting Adeline to take care of him at the expense of herself (Microsystem). It is also apparent that both Adeline and Manny have internalized colonialized, traditional, heteronormative roles despite having both areas of privilege and disadvantage in their backgrounds (macrosystem).

You all explored the influence of culture, acculturation, internalization of privilege, and ways that Manny was moving into a role of having destructive entitlement (despite also being a minority) while Adeline was moving into the role of a martyr under the guise of culture. There was also an exploration of the impact of internalized stereotypes and how the couple wanted to organize their relationship in ways that honored their own voices and loyalty to each other, as well as created generational justice. Through many sessions of ups and downs, therapy seemed to have reorganized their relationship and diminished the tension even after Adeline met Manny's father, despite Manny's father's cut off and estrangement with him because of the relationship. When Adeline and Manny paused treatment, Manny was still in the process of considering repair with his father around the lack of acceptance of his relationship with Adeline.

Lessons from the Chapter

In this chapter, we discussed interracial dating and couple formation and the systemic influences involved (i.e., history, religion, media, family, community, friends, and family). Approval from multiple systemic levels influences these interracial, intercultural, and interfaith couples. What often happens, is that the couple is forced to negotiate family traditions and practices on behalf of family, friends, community, the law, and society while in the beginning stages of dating and throughout their relationship. In evaluating loyalty, fairness/equity, generational messages, and society, interracial and intercultural partners can feel freer to express their relationship boundaries, traditions, and communication around this to others. Extended exercises are included in Appendix 4.1.

Appendix 4.1: Dating and Couple Formation with Your Interracial/Intercultural/Interfaith Clients

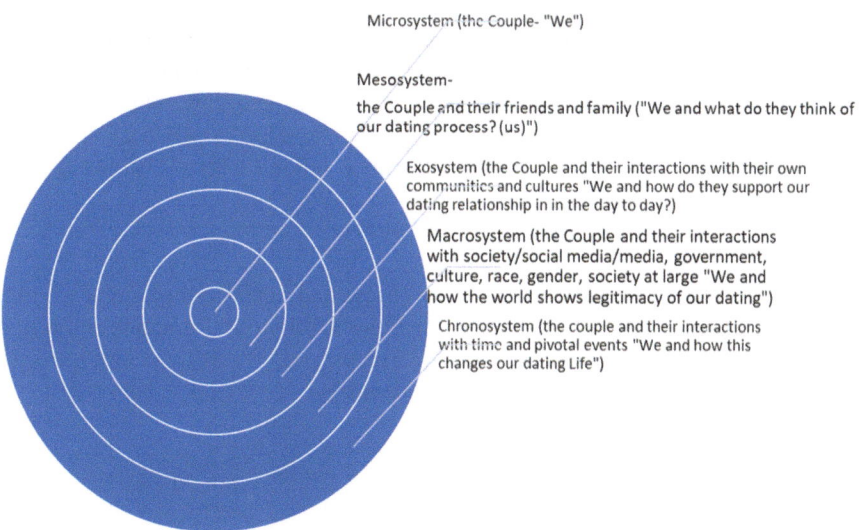

Microsystem (the Couple- "We")

Mesosystem-
the Couple and their friends and family ("We and what do they think of our dating process? (us)")

Exosystem (the Couple and their interactions with their own communities and cultures "We and how do they support our dating relationship in in the day to day?)

Macrosystem (the Couple and their interactions with society/social media/media, government, culture, race, gender, society at large "We and how the world shows legitimacy of our dating")

Chronosystem (the couple and their interactions with time and pivotal events "We and how this changes our dating Life")

The questions below provide a guided reflection across the ecological systems to inform your interventions with interracial and intercultural partners around the topic of dating and couple formation. Please complete this exercise after you have reflected and written down answers from Table 2.1. As you respond to the questions, please consider keywords from Table 2.1. For further exercise, imagine the graphic on this page, as a replacement of the top graphic in Appendix 2.1.

Microsystem—"We"

- What keywords do you notice about the couple's social location and identities in their dating and how they formed their relationship with each other? What keywords/patterns do you see when you consider intersections of privilege/disadvantage?
- What keywords/meaning/stories do you hear when the couple discusses their dating history in relationship to messages and equity when they integrate race, culture, sexuality, gender, or religion?

Mesosystem—"Us"

- What stories, stereotypes, and/or biases do you notice the couple discussing when considering dating and couple formation and their current or previous friends and family influences? How did/will you consider intersections of privilege or disadvantage?
- What levels of approval (positive or negative) does the couple have about culture, race, sexuality, gender, and religion from growing up? (Does this change based upon the life stage of the family members?) How do stories of my interracial, intercultural, or interfaith clients influence their relationship between themselves, their peers, and family members?

Exosystem—"Them"

- What messages do you notice the couple discussing when considering dating and couple formation and their community influences? How did/will you consider intersections of privilege or disadvantage?
- What community messages (positive or negative) do the interracial, intercultural, and interfaith partners have about culture, race, sexuality, gender, and religion from growing up in their communities, previously and currently? (related to humor, specific events, acculturation, trauma, etc.) How do all these stories of my interracial, intercultural, or interfaith clients influence their relationship with the communities that shape them?

Macrosystem—"World"

- What messages from government, advocacy, and social policy influence the interracial, intercultural, and interfaith partner relationship formation and negotiations? How did/will you consider intersections of privilege or disadvantage with the entities you have been associated with?

- How do historical or current laws and policies influence the stories of interracial, intercultural, or interfaith clients?

  Chronosystem—"Life"

- What messages do you notice about the interracial, intercultural, and interfaith partners over the timeline of their relationship in how they address approval, stereotypes, and other macro messages about their relationship? With others?
- How did you consider intersections of privilege or disadvantage with the entities you have been associated with?

References

Addison, S., & Coolhart, D. (2009). Integrating socially segregated identities: Queer couples and the question of race. In M. Rastogi & V. Thomas (Eds.), *Multicultural couple therapy* (pp. 51–75). Sage. https://doi.org/10.4135/9781452275000.n4

Alabama Secretary of State. (n.d.). *Proposed constitutional amendments*. Alabama Votes. https://www.sos.alabama.gov/alabama-votes/voter/election-information/2000/proposed-ammendments

Allen, C. K., & Uskul, A. K. (2019). Preference for dating out-group members: Not the same for all out-groups and cultural backgrounds. *International Journal of Intercultural Relations, 68*, 55–66. https://doi.org/10.1016/j.ijintrel.2018.11.002

Boyd, B., Stephens, D. P., Eaton, A., & Bruk-Lee, V. (2021). Exploring partner scarcity: Highly educated Black women and dating compromise. *Sexuality Research and Social Policy, 18*, 702–714. https://doi.org/10.1007/s13178-020-00493-3

Buggs, S. G. (2017). Does (mixed-) race matter? The role of race in interracial sex, dating, and marriage. *Sociology Compass, 11*(11), 1–13. https://doi.org/10.1111/soc4.12531

Burke, J. L. (2015). Investigating psychological distress in Latino romantic relationships. *Race, Gender & Class, 22*(3–4), 172–194.

Chuang, R., Wilkins, C., Tan, M., & Mead, C. (2021). Racial minorities' attitudes toward interracial couples: An intersection of race and gender. *Group Processes & Intergroup Relations, 24*(3), 453–467. https://doi.org/10.1177/1368430219899482

Csizmadia, A., Leslie, L., & Nazarian, R. (2015). Understanding and treating interracial families. In S. Browning & K. Pasley (Eds.), *Contemporary families: Translating research into practice* (pp. 89–107). Routledge/Taylor & Francis Group.

Cyrus, K. (2017). Multiple minorities as multiply marginalized: Applying the minority stress theory to LGBTQ people of color. *Journal of Gay & Lesbian Mental Health, 21*(3), 194–202.

Field, C. J., Kimuna, S. R., & Straus, M. A. (2013). Attitudes toward interracial relationships among college students: Race, class, gender, and perceptions of parental views. *Journal of Black Studies, 44*(7), 741–776. https://doi.org/10.1177/0021934713507580

Foeman, A., & Nance, T. (2002). Building new cultures, refraining old images: Success strategies of interracial couples. *Howard Journal of Communications, 13*(3), 237–249. https://doi.org/10.1080/10646170290109716

Gilmer, J. A. (2017). *Slavery and freedom in Texas: Stories from the courtroom, 1821–1871* (Vol. 1). University of Georgia Press.

Gonlin, V. (2023). "Come back home, sista!": Reactions to Black women in interracial relationships with White men. *Ethnic and Racial Studies*. https://doi.org/10.1080/01419870.2023.2172353

Guo, M., Li, S., Liu, J., & Sun, F. (2015). Family relations, social connections, and mental health among Latino and Asian older adults. *Research on Aging, 37*(2), 123–147.

Gutierrez, B. C., Halim, M. L. D., & Leaper, C. (2022). Variations in recalled familial messages about gender in relation to emerging adults' gender, ethnic background, and current gender attitudes. *Journal of Family Studies, 28*(1), 150–183. https://doi.org/10.1080/1322940 0.2019.1685562

Harris, T. M., & Kalbfleisch, P. J. (2000). Interracial dating: The implications of race for initiating a romantic relationship. *Howard Journal of Communications, 11*(1), 49–64. https://doi.org/10.1080/106461700246715

Henderson, A. K., & Brantley, M. J. (2019). Parent's just don't understand: Parental support, religion and depressive symptoms among same-race and interracial relationships. *Religions, 10*(3), 1–17.

Hertlein, K., Timm, T. M., & D'Aniello, C. (2020). Integrating couple therapy into work with sexual dysfunctions. In *The handbook of systemic family therapy* (Vol. 3–4, pp. 363–383). Wiley-Blackwell. https://doi.org/10.1002/9781119438519.ch75

James, J. G., Coard, S. I., Fine, M. A., & Rudy, D. (2018). The central roles of race and racism in reframing family systems theory: A consideration of choice and time. *Journal of Family Theory & Review, 10*(2), 419–433. https://doi.org/10.1111/jftr.12262

Jordan, S. N. (2019). *White parents, mixed race children: The entangled effects of love, racism, and parenting* (Publication No. 345088574) [Doctoral dissertation, Appalachian State University]. CORE.

Lundquist, J. H., & Lin, K. H. (2015). Is love (color) blind? The economy of race among gay and straight daters. *Social Forces, 93*(4), 1423–1449. https://doi.org/10.1093/SF/SOV008

Mayer, C., & Viviers, R. (2017). Experiences of shame by race and culture: An exploratory study. *Journal of Psychology in Africa, 27*(4), 362–366. https://doi.org/10.1080/1433023 7.2017.1347759

McGrath, A. R., Tsunokai, G. T., Schultz, M., Kavanagh, J., & Tarrence, J. A. (2016). Differing shades of colour: Online dating preferences of biracial individuals. *Ethnic and Racial Studies, 39*(11), 1920–1942. https://doi.org/10.1080/01419870.2015.1131313

Morales, E. (2012). Parental messages concerning Latino/Black interracial dating: An exploratory study among Latina/o young adults. *Latino Studies, 10*(3), 314–333. https://doi.org/10.1057/lst.2012.24

Muro, J., & Martinez, L. (2016). Constrained desires: The romantic partner preferences of college-educated Latinas. *Latin American Research Review, 14*, 172–191. https://doi.org/10.1057/lst.2016.3

Perry, S. L. (2014). Hoping for a Godly (White) family: How desire for religious heritage affects whites' attitudes toward interracial marriage. *Journal for the Scientific Study of Religion, 53*(1), 202–218. https://doi.org/10.1111/jssr.12079

Prasad, P. (2018). More color more pride: Addressing structural barriers to interracial LGBTQ loving. *Fordham Law Review Online, 87*, 89–100.

Ranzini, G., & Rosenbaum, J. E. (2020). It's a match (?): Tinder usage and attitudes toward interracial dating. *Communication Research Reports, 37*(1–2), 44–54. https://doi.org/10.108 0/08824096.2020.1748001

Riley, N. S. (2013). *'Til faith do us part: How interfaith marriage is transforming America*. Oxford University Press.

Robinson, B. A. (2015). "Personal preference" as the new racism: Gay desire and racial cleansing in cyberspace. *Sociology of Race and Ethnicity, 1*(2), 317–330.

Rosenfeld, M. J., & Kim, B. S. (2005). The independence of young adults and the rise of interracial and same-sex unions. *American Sociological Review, 70*(4), 541–562.

Simpson, G. E., & Yinger, J. M. (2013). *Racial and cultural minorities: An analysis of prejudice and discrimination*. Springer Science & Business Media.

Stein, G. L., Gonzalez, L. M., Cupito, A. M., Kiang, L., & Supple, A. J. (2015). The protective role of familism in the lives of Latino adolescents. *Journal of Family Issues, 36*(10), 1255–1273.

Steinbugler, A. C. (2005). Visibility as privilege and danger: Heterosexual and same-sex interracial intimacy in the 21st century. *Sexualities, 8*(4), 425–443.

Wu, K., Chen, C., & Greenberger, E. (2015). The sweetness of forbidden fruit: Interracial daters are more attractive than intraracial daters. *Journal of Social and Personal Relationships, 32*(5), 650–666. https://doi.org/10.1177/0265407514541074

Zhou, Z. B. (2022). Compulsory interracial intimacy: Why does removing the ethnicity filter on dating apps not benefit racial minorities? *Media, Culture & Society, 44*(5), 1034–1043. https://doi.org/10.1177/01634437221104712

Chapter 5
Interracial and Intercultural Cohabitation: How Do We Share Space Emotionally and Physically?

> *...And learning differences, different preferences, or ways of growing up because his upbringing is different than mine. You know, I understand the differences and that it's not wrong, it's just different. Sometimes very different.*
>
> ~Vanessa, (Kalnasy, 2015, p. 60)

Cohabitation: Not Just Us

Previously, in US culture, the stereotypic romantic sequence was linear: dating > engagement > cohabitation > marriage > children; now demographers have been documenting that this pattern is no longer the norm, nor even linear, and children often precede marriage, cohabitation, and even engagement with intraracial (monoracial) couples. Cohabitation has increased within recent decades, with more than half of adults, aged 18–44, having lived with an unmarried partner and 78% of young adults, aged 18–29, reporting it is acceptable for cohabitation before marriage (Pew Research Center, 2019). Another study from 2017, reported 18% of cohabiting adults identified as interracial/intercultural (Livingston, 2017), and research has shown that interracial and intercultural couples cohabitate at lower rates than the general population (Choi et al., 2022). This may be due to cultural or religious values that strongly oppose cohabitation before marriage and even having a sexual relationship.

In many cultures, sex and sexuality are intertwined with tradition and familial bonds, particularly around religiosity. However, religion is starting to become detached from this process. For example, 89% of Single Christians surveyed voiced that they were not planning to and didn't want to wait for marriage to have sex; 77% didn't need love for sex, only 40% said that they wouldn't engage in casual sex, and 95% would not wait for an engagement to have sex. As collectivist cultures largely prioritize familial and social approval, which may include religion, cohabitating before marriage may cause internalized distress and identity conflict and interfere with commitment. However, couples who cohabitate (both interracial and monoracial) have also reported a sense of independence, relationship identity development, and stability in marriage (Sassler, 2004). Thus, even before living together,

© American Family Therapy Academy (AFTA) 2024
G. Seshadri, D. Gutierrez, *Interracial, Intercultural, and Interfaith Couples and Families Across the Life Cycle*, AFTA SpringerBriefs in Family Therapy, https://doi.org/10.1007/978-3-031-58538-8_5

differences in support or opposition to cohabitation, family and cultural values, intercultural relational identity negotiation, and intrapersonal identity expression are processes that interracial/intercultural partnerships may need to navigate.

It is important for clinicians to probe how the interracial partners feel about living together; if they have opposition from family and friends based on cultural rules or religious rules and how this impacts their community presence. In addition, probing for feelings about marriage or if marriage is a goal is important to explore. Often interracial and intercultural partners may have to not only hide their relationship but may also have to hide their cohabitation from friends and family, leading to even more isolation. With isolation, there may be more emotional pressure between partners than in intraracial relationships. Some interracial and intercultural partners will not move in together without the promise of engagement.

For example, Sabina (cisgender, South Asian female, immigrant parents) would not agree to move in with Taylor (transgender, Asian, male-identifying—they/them pronouns, immigrant parents) until they proposed. This created a subtle tension, as the couple had been together for almost 10 years and Sabina's family still viewed Taylor as Sabina's "friend." Prior to Taylor's gender-affirming hormone therapy and surgery, Taylor and Sabina lived together as Sabina's "roommate"; and now they do not, as Taylor has already transitioned and presents as male. Living together before marriage goes against Sabina's family culture. Previously and now, the family was aware of Taylor's presence, but not as a romantic partner, which often makes Taylor feel left out. According to Taylor's chosen family (Taylor is estranged from their family of origin due to a lack of support), Taylor still faces discomfort when bringing Sabina around, because of how Sabina's family has treated them. A clinician working with the couple might help them navigate how to create shared space between them emotionally to support each other with each other's families (chosen and biological). For example, hearing each other out and finding a way to address feelings of invisibility for both, so they both feel acknowledged and that they belong. The clinician would also need to explore how to share space physically in the loss of Sabina's familial bond, without it taking a toll on the couple's commitment to each other and honoring both their values and cultures. The clinician might even intermittently invite Taylor's chosen family to sessions as a form of support for both partners.

Mesosystem and Moving Towards Sharing: Day-to-Day Navigation

Although there are individual microsystems in the relationship, an interracial/intercultural couple's environments and interactions blend. Their cultural identity as a couple could be considered their mesosystem. As a couple, alone, decision-making processes of cohabitation are no longer solely around attraction, getting to know someone, and physically separate individualistic lifestyles, but now involve finances, family expansion, increased sexual communication, religious ritual preferences, and discussion of marriage. Essentially, the partners must discover how to collaborate in these shared spaces.

For same-race couples, barriers around race/ethnicity/culture/traditions/family approval are usually nonexistent, because the focus is not on negotiating differences and expectations or other opportunities for microaggressions, or even celebrating their love, because they haven't violated any social expectations (Campbell & Martin, 2016). More specifically, "family opposition tends to be stronger for interracial marriage than for interracial cohabitation" (as cited by Choi et al., 2022, p. 958). Despite minimal research and literature on the stability and longevity of interracial cohabitation, it has been suggested that race is the biggest impediment in marriage (Choi et al., 2022). However, since most interracial couple research has been done on Black-White couples, we do not know of cohabitation statistics with other interracial combinations and the influence of race on them or other cultural factors. Thus, considering the intersectionality of the partners' social locations, clinicians need to be aware of how interracial and intercultural dynamics may play out in shared living spaces. For example, WOC not being paid as much and may not be able to afford a house/separate housing before marriage due to economic conditions and gender considerations (Nicola et al., 2020). Clinicians need to be aware of complicated dynamics and ask themselves how intersectionality will play a role.

On the other hand, some interracial couples may see cohabitation as a nonthreatening way to be together as they navigate life transitions connected to culture and race (Choi et al., 2022). Though cohabitating may be seen as a negative or less preferred transition based on societal and religious ideals and cultural stigma related to sex and commitment, it can also help interracial and intercultural couples create stability and a strong foundation for a long-term relationship in which they are able to navigate life cycles and shifts that can weather racial and cultural differences.

For example, socioeconomic status (SES) is an evident form of a life cycle change through blending and pooling resources. Contextually, interracial/intercultural couples potentially need to navigate an additional layer of financial distress that same race, and particularly same race, White couples, don't face. Interracial couples with White, Hispanic, and Black partners tend to hold less privilege, as do partners who are immigrants and less assimilated (Choi et al., 2022; Choi & Tienda, 2017). However, generations of migration (first generation to fourth generation) may also impact SES, access to opportunities or income, or financial values. For example, a couple comprised of Susan (White, cisgender, heterosexual female, raised in lower middle SES) and Xander (Asian, cisgender, heterosexual male, raised in upper SES, third generation) may never had a conversation on finances before deciding to move in together. One major financial burden today involves student loans. Susan had to take out a significant amount for academia, while Xander was able to have his family take care of tuition. As Susan and Xander have begun to search for homes, Susan's financial debt limits their home-buying potential, a financial limitation that Xander may not have experienced. Despite education normally being viewed as privilege, in this way, it can also be a form of disadvantage that can create conflict and impact the balance of power between partners.

A therapist you could guide Susan and Xander to discuss their financial values and experiences and how, as a couple, they would negotiate this aspect of their relationship. Questions might include: When do you have discussions on finances as a couple? What are your cultural values around family of origin and money? Individually, how did you manage your own finances and what did it mean to you to manage your finances at the time? Did this change when you started to cohabitate? Did your parents or caregivers talk openly about finances while you were growing up? Identity differences are also evident, as Xander's family has financial status and expects education as a path to success from their Asian immigrant experience, while Susan's family, centered family roles and financial responsibilities to manage a home day to day as an accomplishment. Further discussion of these values, SES, and power inequity may raise discomfort and nuance regarding how they will manage their expenses, but will ultimately bring the couple to mutual understanding of buying, maintaining, and sustaining resources together.

Historical Exosystem Impact: Multiple Intersecting Identity Cohabitation and Navigation

Little research has focused on cohabitation and couplings of various intersecting sexual, racial, and gender identities. Just 70 years ago, "homosexuality" was categorized as a "sociopathic personality disturbance" and was criminalized in the United States at the same time as racial segregation and brutality. Any form of intersecting identity coupling was not only frowned upon but could result in death; keeping these unions secretive was necessary for safety (Rosenfeld & Kim, 2005). It is important to note that despite authors discussing the isolation and feelings of loneliness from being hidden and lack of support as interracial and intercultural couples, and while literature has compared the coming out of an interracial, interracial, and interfaith couple to that of an LGBTQ+ member's coming process, there are nuances and differences between these processes despite them appearing or being associated as similar.

Only 12 years ago "Don't ask, don't tell" was repealed, which banned sexually diverse individuals from serving in the military, while simultaneously, systemic and entrenched racism was and still is persistent in armed forces (Rogin, 2021). Same-sex marriage was legalized nationwide only 8 years ago (Lee, 2018), and both same-sex and interracial marriage were codified in federal law and finally protected from overturn in the United States through the Respect for Marriage Act (H.R.8404, 2022). Before these laws came into effect, same-sex interracial and intercultural partners had only the option to cohabitate and lacked legal benefits (and protections) of marriage.

Despite these efforts, continued and increased anti-LGBTQ legislation is evident. Already in 2023, a staggering 318 bills were introduced and 21 enacted against the rights and safety of LGBTQ+ community, creating more fear and unrest (American Civil Liberties Union [ACLU], 2024). Moreover, accounts of these societal stressors still tend to center around sexually and gender-diverse communities and lack of understanding of dual, multifaceted experiences. Sexually and gender-diverse communities still center on White experiences. Intersections of ethnicity, race, sexuality, and gender are left out in research, clinical work, and legislation. When working with LGBTQ+ interracial, intercultural, and/or interfaith partners, it is important to explore these intersections. Ask questions such as: How does the recent legislation influence you? How does this influence your community within your home, neighborhood, and community? How do these societal impacts affect you?

Cohabitation may impact individual and relational identities in various ways; for example, being able to be in partnership(s) as one's individual and relational identity grow may provide safety and decrease minority stressors (Frost & Meyer, 2009). Also, cohabitation with partners can involve a rich and diverse network of relationships, such as parents, grandparents, extended family, siblings, and chosen families; all of whom influence relational development. Each of these circles of influence can also offer support to interracial and intercultural partners.

Other contextual factors such as lack of acceptance from family members, decreased finances, and lack of community may all be factors contributing to cohabitation. There are higher instances of same-sex interracial couples in metropolitan cities, where acceptance and support for their identities are more prominent than in rural townships (Grether & Jones, 2021). However, and interestingly enough, interracial same-sex relationships are more likely to cohabitate today than different sex same race couples (i.e., heterosexual relationships) (Schwartz & Graf, 2009). Evidence may also be scarce because sexually, ethnically, and gender-diverse couples may have not reported or shared cohabiting status in fear and distress around lack of overall societal acceptance (Moore et al., 2015). This can influence the lack of research, creating unknowns regarding intersecting racial and ethnic factors.

Engagement and Marriages: Navigating Cultural and Religious Differences

A few studies show that education and economic status were greatly linked to willingness to intermarry. However, our deep dive search in various search engines using the words "engagement" and "wedding planning" coupled with "interracial," "intercultural," and "interfaith" yielded search results of only six books and no articles or other sources. When looking up the words engagement, wedding planning, etc., resources abound involved in navigating cultural norms and traditions (i.e., interracial, intercultural, and interfaith), K1 visa process (immigration laws and regulations), wedding planning, and Christian interracial marriage or Christian and Jewish interfaith marriage. However, these sources were limited in generalizing to interracial combinations or interfaith relationships. Even premarital assessments using issues relevant to interracial couples are minimal and don't address cultural or interfaith issues; rather they appear to lump interracial and intercultural couples with the same assessments as same-race couples (Wong, 2009).

Macrosystem/Exosystem

This highlights the lack of support (macrosystemically and exosystemically) in peer-reviewed research or a simple Google search in helping interracial and intercultural couples navigate important life transitions. If race, culture, and faith are all big navigations, why aren't there more strength-based sources on how to navigate them? What happens if a couple announces their engagement, and their family estranges or cuts off from them? This estrangement can become a developmental struggle/stressor for the couple and can impact repair with the family if damage feels irreconcilable (mesosystemically). Here a therapist could dive into cultural differences around desires or expectations around family, engagement, and marriage; processes that may not have been unearthed before. Questions such as "What messages did you receive about marriage and family when you were growing up? Tell me about strengths you have within your relationship? how can we translate these strengths to nurture distress from family cut-off?" can be used to emphasize a need to communicate and support one another, rather than internalizing the distress. With familial acceptance, time (chronosystem) and mutual ways of relating to each other can help transcend barriers to acceptance of their interracial, intercultural, and/or interfaith union (Seshadri & Knudson-Martin, 2013). Same-sex partners or those identifying as nonbinary, queer, or other minority statuses may face the additional burden of finding businesses to perform services that support their unions.

The goal of this phase of life (i.e., engagement or marriage speculation) is to celebrate and honor the couple and their families and help the couple decide how to best honor them based on their relationship structure, that is, whether they organize around culture through integration, singular assimilation, or co-existing, rather than one-size-fits-all "shoulds" (Seshadri & Knudson-Martin, 2013). Ceremonially, this may look like integrating both sets of traditions (integrated), only showcasing one partner's traditions (singularly assimilated), or having two separate ceremonies (co-existing). With sexually and gender-diverse couples, traditions are often steeped in patriarchy and heteronormativity, so a couple may have to create their own version of wedding traditions meaningful to them (Arend, 2016).

Negotiating and creating a couple's own rules can be a potential strategy for interracial and intercultural couples to use in an already stressful process of wedding planning. Overall, through meso- (e.g., family/friends/neighbors), macro- (e.g., community and businesses), exo- (e.g., the law), and chronosystemic levels (e.g., over time), a couple can communicate their couple identity both individually and systemically through meaning and language. For further awareness and suggested exercises, please refer to Appendix 5.1.

Narrative Deconstruction/Reconstruction

To incorporate a strength-based perspective we return to social constructionism and ecological systems theory. Social constructionism focuses on understanding relationships, social action, and language as a product of the times (Gergen & Gergen, 2003). With this ecological, social constructionist lens, the meaning and messages behind race, culture, and marriage capture societal influences on the couple and the couple identity and reflect reciprocal processes between society and the development of the couple identity. This perspective will enable a focus on how interracial couples create meaningful relationships and provide a theoretical framework for understanding what works to build and sustain these marriages to help them thrive.

One clinical goal is to focus on creating a foundation for the partners, (i.e., a cohabitation identity). This can comprise the relationship identity, but also can be an identity or a plan that incorporates other aspects such as finances, chores of living together, and integration of tradition. Since relationship identity is socially constructed, emotions are a part of the relationship rather than simply an individual experience. Since partners share emotional space, how emotional support is given and shared needs to be also a part of the cohabitation identity.

It is also important to deconstruct family approval, regardless of whether partners are gender fluid, same-sex, or male/female. Often, values from the families of origin can threaten partners, especially if the family is not supportive due to misalignment with cultural values. If so, partners will need emotional support and understanding from each other, a discussion of boundaries between family members and the partners, and perhaps a plan around estrangement if this is threatened. Sometimes families don't distinguish between cultural traditions and behaviors they were raised with. Or perhaps they don't know much about the interracial/intercultural/interfaith partner and make assumptions about their inability to relate to them. Lack of family support can also be connected to expectations and/or the immigrant/American dream.

For example, parents can put pressure on a particular interracial partner (Paul, cisgender male, Native American) to move out of the reservation, get a house, and propose to their child, Laura (cisgender female, Hispanic), instead of living together, while Paul is going through school. They believe this as a function of their values and the immigrant dream (getting married, buying a house, having children, and being released of responsibility of Laura, etc.). They may threaten estrangement from Laura because of these expectations not being met. Both Paul and Laura need to decide how much parental approval means to them and choose how much contact to have with Laura's parents. The clinician must help with this process, through validation, action planning, and continual assessment of emotional support between partners and others.

Normativity

Secondly, we must discuss the role of normativity, in all aspects; racial, sexual orientation, gender, and culture. This applies not only to same-sex partners but also nonbinary and male/female cisgender partners. More specifically, in cohabitation the clinician needs to be skilled at asking questions that challenge normative views to figure out what works for the couple; are they doing it because it's normative for others based on culture, class, gender, sex, etc.? Another question to ask is if we do this in a normative way, how is that helpful to us? Will it harm us in any way or make our identity invisible? If we choose to do things differently, what is the benefit and how can it cost us both financially and emotionally?

It is also important to explore if the couple wants marriage or is in preparation for marriage. This doesn't always mean that there is a proposal and engagement. If the couple wants to move towards marriage, what are some traditions and practices that they want to engage in? How do they want to involve others? If this involves family or lack thereof, how will this impact their finances? What do our values want to be around money? How have our previous financial decisions, both individually and as a couple, going to affect us? Additionally, religion, and sometimes even spirituality, can be very prescriptive; clinicians serve clients best in having conversations around how the partners want to engage this relationship both individually and as a couple and how this might factor in, in regard to tradition, and if the couple decides to celebrate their relationship through marriage. For example, if they are meeting with a religious leader, could they even acknowledge that they were living together before marriage, much less having a sexual relationship because they wanted to explore sexual compatibility? And how much would the religious leader and family be involved in the relationship problems of the couple? All these aspects of the life stage of preparing for marriage are ripe for opportunities to explore that will help create an identity and foundation for the couple.

Lastly, sometimes, the assumption for a cohabitating partnership is that they are making individual decisions while living under the same roof, or that they are "waiting to co-mingle" things like finances until after marriage. Or that the couple sees themselves as individual partners because they are cohabitating. It is important that clinicians probe for this, as there may be different internalized rules for cohabitation that are informed by culture, family of origin, or even faith. An additional reframe in these situations would be to reframe cohabitation as creating a foundation for the future.

Opening culture and religion for discussion offers multiple possibilities and options for how to relate to it. When two or more cultures intermix through marriage or a significant relationship, questions surface as to how stories and traditions "should be" followed and how differences "should be" addressed. They need to create a set of shared beliefs and experiences that is a reality to them. Shared values and holding on to special customs or traditions can help to preserve the couple's relationship.

Case Application

You once saw a couple who came in to discuss lack of communication and romance within their relationship. Maria identified as Latina, cisgender female, lesbian woman, and her partner Leslie was White, trans male, pansexual. During the pandemic, their lives had gone from independence to complete and total integration of their lives when they decided to move in together after 5 months of dating. Leslie said he felt emasculated by Maria at times taking the brunt of her angry outbursts, which would bring up internalized gender minority stressors that he had worked on in the past but have been building recently. "She has no idea how I literally crumble up inside when she yells and gets so angry, no way can I be the man she desires when I am the man she attacks." Maria also felt disempowered by Leslie when he becomes tired of loud music and constant facetiming with her parents and grandparents. "He is literally disrespecting me and my culture, why would I want to be romantic or even talk with him?" (quotes edited for anonymity).

As you hear them go back and forth with one another, their yelling begins to escalate, enough so that after the session your colleague comes to check if you were okay. You acknowledge that you felt lost in the overwhelming contextual and systemic premises occurring in their relationship. You could also imagine how lost they felt too, and all while navigating a global pandemic. You begin with this thought in their next session (after being glad/nervous they came back). Through a narrative lens, you all begin to deconstruct language that has been thrown around in arguments, conversation, or even in thought. They started with "lost," feelings of loss surrounded not only being systemically caught in the weeds but also microsystemically with their own freedoms. The freedom for Maria to go to her mom's house and eat her favorite dish arroz con *habichuela y pollo*. The freedom for Leslie to go to his friends' houses and have game nights. Loss then came in what they expected their relationship to be, mesosystemically, once they moved in together. The fun and laughter they had 100% of the time they had spent together dwindled once conversations about rent, space, and vulnerability occurred. Maria felt a relational loss of Leslie's respect and love of her culture.

Leslie had not realized that asking Maria to "turn down" these pieces of her life was essentially toning down what pieces of culture she was grasping to keep. Maria had not realized that her behavior was toning down Leslie's masculinity journey, which he also grasped at during this overall time of loss. Once Leslie and Maria were able to grieve their micro and meso losses, we were able to reauthor their narrative as individuals and as a couple. They included one another in their music, family calls, culture, and identity journeys and shifted from reactive, defensive responses to shared, responsive responses.

Lessons from the Chapter

In this chapter, we discussed interracial cohabitation and the systemic influences involved in sharing physical space (i.e., housing, daily activities, chores) and emotional space with each other (i.e., finances, marriage preparation and traditions, family members' approval/disapproval). Often what happens is that the couple is forced to negotiate family traditions and practices on behalf of family, friends, community, the law and society, and the quagmire of cultural and religious traditions. In deconstructing and reconstructing meaningful traditions for the couple, the interracial and intercultural partners can feel freer to express their relationship boundaries, traditions, and communication around each other and to others. Extended exercises are included in Appendix 5.1.

Appendix 5.1: Cohabitation and Pre-marriage with Your Interracial/Intercultural/Interfaith Clients

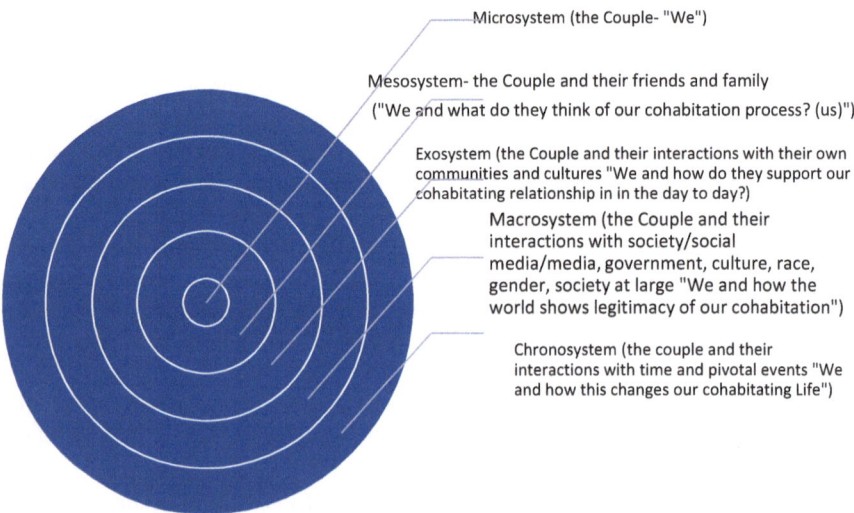

The questions below provide a guided reflection across the ecological systems to inform your interventions with interracial and intercultural partners around the topic of cohabitation and marriage preparation. Please complete this exercise after you have reflected and written down answers from Table 2.1. As you respond to the questions, please consider keywords from Table 2.1. For further exercise, imagine the graphic on this page, as a replacement of the top graphic in Appendix 2.1.

Microsystem—"We"

- What keywords do you notice about the couple's social location and identities in their discussions of cohabitation, discussion of chores and responsibilities, and/ or marriage preparation?
- What keywords or patterns do you see when you consider intersections of privilege or disadvantage?
- What keywords/meaning do you hear when the couple discusses how they manage chores and responsibilities, and possibilities around marriage? How do they negotiate normativity with them when they integrate race, culture, sexuality, gender, or religion?

Mesosystem—"Us"

- What stories or messages do you notice the couple discussing when considering cohabitation, finances, shared space, and their current or previous friends and family influence?
- How did/will you consider intersections of privilege or disadvantage?
- What levels of approval (positive or negative) does the couple have about culture, race, sexuality, gender, and religion from growing up? (Does this change based on the life stage of the family members?) How is this influenced by cohabitation? Traditions?

Exosystem—"Them"

- What messages do you notice the couple discussing when considering finances, cohabitation, chores, and their community influence? How did/will you consider intersections of privilege or disadvantage?
- What community messages (positive or negative) do the interracial, intercultural, and interfaith partners have about culture, race, sexuality, gender, and religion from growing up in their communities, previously and currently in relationship to finances and cohabitation? (related to humor, specific events, acculturation, trauma, etc.)
- How do all these stories of my interracial, intercultural, or interfaith clients influence their relationships and the communities that shape them?

Macrosystem—"World"

- What messages from government, advocacy, and social policy influence the interracial, intercultural, and interfaith partners around cohabitation, finances, or chores?
- How did you consider intersections of privilege or disadvantage with the entities you have been associated with?
- How do historical or current laws and policies, influence the stories of the interracial, intercultural, or interfaith clients around cohabitation, finances, or chores?

Chronosystem—"Life"

- What messages do you notice about the interracial, intercultural, and interfaith partners over the timeline of their relationship in how they address approval, division of labor, and other macro messages about their relationship? With others?
- How did/will you consider intersections of privilege or disadvantage with the entities you have been associated with?
- How do they address bias, stereotypes, and other macro messages about their relationship? With others?

References

American Civil Liberties Union. (2024, January 19). *Mapping attacks on LGBTQ rights in the U.S. state legislatures in 2024.* https://www.aclu.org/legislative-attacks-on-lgbtq-rights-2024

Arend, P. (2016). Consumption as common sense: Heteronormative hegemony and white wedding desire. *Journal of Consumer Culture, 16*(1), 144–163.

Campbell, M. E., & Martin, M. A. (2016). Race, immigration and exogamy among the native born: Variation across communities. *Sociology of Race and Ethnicity, 2*, 142–161. https://doi.org/10.1177/2332649215598786

Choi, K. H., & Tienda, M. (2017). Marriage-market constraints and mate-selection behavior: Racial, ethnic, and gender differences in intermarriage. *Journal of Marriage and the Family, 79*(2), 301–317. https://doi.org/10.1111/jomf.12346

Choi, K. H., Goldberg, R. E., & Denice, P. A. (2022). Stability and outcome of interracial cohabitation before and after transitions to marriage. *Demographic Research, 46*, 957–1006. https://doi.org/10.4054/DemRes.2022.46.33

Frost, D. M., & Meyer, I. H. (2009). Internalized homophobia and relationship quality among lesbians, gay men, and bisexuals. *Journal of Counseling Psychology, 56*(1), 97–109. https://doi.org/10.1037/a0012844

Gergen, M., & Gergen, K. J. (2003). Marriage as a relational engagement. *Feminism & Psychology, 13*(4), 469–474. https://doi.org/10.1177/09593535030134012

Grether, S. T., & Jones, A. (2021). Examining the relationship between social support and interracial divorce in Louisiana. *Journal of Family Issues, 42*(8), 1831–1851. https://doi.org/10.1177/0192513X20957363

H.R.8404—117th Congress (2021–2022): Respect for Marriage Act. (2022, December 13). https://www.congress.gov/bill/117th-congress/house-bill/8404

Kalnasy, M. L. (2015). Fighting the Stereotypes: How Black-White Interracial Couples Strengthen and Maintain their Relationships (Order No. 3668670). Available from ProQuest Dissertations & Theses Global; Publicly Available Content Database. (1648413367). https://www.0-search.proquest.com.library.alliant.edu/dissertations-theses/fightingstereotypes-how-black-white-interracial/docview/1648413367/se-2

Lee, J. (2018). Black LGB identities and perceptions of same-sex marriage. *Journal of Homosexuality, 65*(14), 2005–2027. https://doi.org/10.1080/00918369.2017.1423214

Livingston, G. (2017, June 8). *Among U.S. cohabiters, 18% have a partner of a different race or ethnicity.* Pew Research Center. Retrieved from https://www.pewresearch.org/short-reads/2017/06/08/among-u-s-cohabiters-18-have-a-partner-of-a-different-race-or-ethnicity/

Moore, J., Kienzle, J., & Flood Grady, E. (2015). Discursive Struggles of Tradition and Nontradition in the Retrospective Accounts of Married Couples Who Cohabited Before Engagement. *Journal of Family Communication, 15*(2), 95–112. https://doi.org/10.1080/15267431.2015.1013109

Nicola, M., Alsafi, Z., Sohrabi, C., Kerwan, A., Al-Jabir, A., Iosifidis, C., Agha, M., & Agha, R. (2020). The socio-economic implications of the coronavirus pandemic (COVID-19): A review. *International Journal of Surgery (London, England), 78*, 185–193. https://doi.org/10.1016/j.ijsu.2020.04.018

Pew Research Center. (2019, November 6). *Marriage and cohabitation in the U.S.* Retrieved from https://www.pewresearch.org/social-trends/2019/11/06/marriage-and-cohabitation-in-the-u-s/#:~:text=Young%20adults%20are%20particularly%20accepting,age%20groups%20share%20this%20view

Rogin, A. (2021). How Don't Ask, Don't Tell has affected LGBTQ service members, 10 years after repeal. *PBS Newshour.* https://www.pbs.org/newshour/nation/how-dont-ask-dont-tell-has-affected-lgbtq-service-members-10-years-after-repeal

Rosenfeld, M. J., & Kim, B. S. (2005). The independence of young adults and the rise of interracial and same-sex unions. *American Sociological Review, 70*(4), 541–562. https://doi.org/10.1177/000312240507000401

Sassler, S. (2004). The process of entering into cohabiting unions. Journal of Marriage and Family, 66(2), 491–505. https://doi.org/10.1111/j.1741-3737.2004.00033.x.

Seshadri, G., & Knudson-Martin, C. (2013). How couples manage interracial and intercultural differences: implications for clinical practice. *Journal of marital and family therapy, 39*(1), 43–58. https://doi.org/10.1111/j.1752-0606.2011.00262.x

Schwartz, C. R., & Graf, N. L. (2009). Assortative matching among same-sex and different-sex couples in the United States, 1990–2000. *Demographic Research, 21*, 843.

Wong, M. K. (2009). Strengthening connections in interracial marriages through pre-marital inventories: A critical literature review. *Contemporary Family Therapy, 31*(4), 251–261. https://doi.org/10.1007/s10591-009-9099-1

Chapter 6
Exploring the "Rules" of Interracial Relationships: Marriage, Nonmonogamy, and Children

I don't believe in rules. Rules are about trying to wall off an insecurity. When I'm triggered, it inspires me to ask where the insecurity is coming from.

Kevin, (Patterson, 2018) PolyRoleModels.tumblr.com

Marriage itself is not an individual endeavor, but a multi-relational one. This is where considerable tension may arise for interracial, intercultural, and interfaith couples. In this chapter, we examine how couples negotiate rules, roles, and issues stemming from their families of origin, and how these apply to nonmonogamy, fertility, pregnancy, and children and parenting.

Mesosystems and Family Marriages

In Western culture, marriage is usually seen as a coupling of "two" people in a union that is "holy matrimony." Then those two people go on with their lives together as their "own" family. However, marriage also means merging families, tradition, culture, language, and customs; each needs to be valued and honored (Greif & Saviet, 2020). Jokes abound about how when one enters marriage, they enter into bed with at least five other people; their parents, their spouse, and their spouse's parents and siblings (i.e., in-laws). Partners may feel the need to legitimize their spouses to their families to help make their partners feel accepted or families may fear their children are experiencing discrimination (Greif & Saviet, 2020; Rockquemore & Henderson, 2010). While partners may hope that their families are as open-minded as they are, laws can also be a source of prejudice, discrimination, and microaggressions.

Clinically, many interracial, intercultural, and interfaith partners have shared with us that while on the surface family members claim to be open, modern, and accepting, they often act in ways that show biases, microaggressions, prejudice, and discrimination through comments, actions, and support of various political policies that impact interracial, intercultural, and interfaith families. Conversations may also be sensitive around what children may look like, including physical features and

© American Family Therapy Academy (AFTA) 2024
G. Seshadri, D. Gutierrez, *Interracial, Intercultural, and Interfaith Couples and Families Across the Life Cycle*, AFTA SpringerBriefs in Family Therapy, https://doi.org/10.1007/978-3-031-58538-8_6

skin color or disagreements around ethnic names. Clinicians need to help navigate conversations about this, even if unartfully brought up by a family member.

While marriage is a celebration of union, families of interracial/intercultural couples face diverse emotions from joy to experiences with racial and structural inequalities, and potential internalized racism of self-worth when marrying someone of another race and culture. Rockquemore and Henderson (2010) provided a narrative of a White male being married to a WOC and racially discriminatory practices he had developed and was unlearning and recognizing when he was using jokes, microaggressions, and comments that were biased/racist. After reflecting and deeper awareness, he no longer participates in these regarding anyone.

Culturally, families share and intergenerationally pass down messages regarding values of marriage and structure. These values are foundational to how family members understand, share, and grow in identity development. With a society based on colonialism and structural oppression, diverse communities have centuries of racial identity development and socialization experience that have formed means of protection for their spouses and children. In his exploration of family of origin and interracial spouses' racial histories and experiences and the impact of silencing painful histories, Killian (2001) found that with a strong history of oppression, discrimination, and violence, families often don't want to "turn back" and ask about race or identity development, particularly for couples with White spouses.

What Do Clinicians Do?

Recognizing potential histories or messages of racism, microaggressions, or intersected sexism is a place of intervention; although potentially a vulnerable one. If working with the couple from the quote above (we will call them Andy and Keena), space would need to be created for Andy to recognize a history of racially discriminatory words or actions and a space for Keena to respond to that history. They would need to explicitly communicate and develop the ability to grow into cultural humility as a couple. Together, they would need to discuss boundaries (i.e., how much others could be let into their world) and responses to any forms of discrimination and how they would overcome them by considering physical and emotional safety.

Even when spouses are both diverse, strong familial messages can create tension within their marriage and from their families. Parents in interracial marriages may have potential fears and protective attitudes toward their children. Changes from a cohesive family of origin to navigating and involving another culture in the family may be a source of tension. Change can have a profound impact on family systems, especially when strong cultural ideologies and bonds are involved; a family may do and say all they can to keep their adult children to who they *know*, rather than who they are *becoming* within their marriages.

A Culture of Silence

A "culture of silence" refers to a phenomenon in families and communities where specific issues, experiences, or histories are deemed "unspeakable" (Amoateng-Boahen, 2015). These topics are avoided in discussion and disclosure of the unspeakable is discouraged. For many families, there are many reasons silence is preferred over discussion. This could include trauma, traditional beliefs and values, and a reluctance to reopen intergenerational wounds over opening Pandora's box and not knowing how to address it. As seen in the quote, these topics may involve sexual violence, estrangement, intergenerational conflicts, or familial struggles.

However, silence negatively impacts individual and relational lives through mental health, identity development and growth, availability of support systems, and challenges to open communication. Silencing processes directed toward maintaining a family's name and reputation may heavily impact adult children's marriages and create tension between who is primary—family of origin or their spouses. Communication may also be impacted through lack of emotional expression, understanding, or knowing how to come to resolution. When spouses are unable to learn these processes in their families of origin, these patterns may continue in their marriages. As with Andy and Keena, if they keep their pain silent within their relationship or their families, that pain would overshadow and hinder their ability as a couple to grow in communication, cultural understanding of one another and their families, and values to pass down to future generations. In effect, this would be a secret that would and could turn into generational trauma.

Spouses must learn how to break and renegotiate patterns of silence through promotion of acceptance, support, sharing, opening dialogue with family members, and challenging cultural norms. A clinician can help facilitate this process by gently exploring generational histories in relationship to race, culture, class, trauma, and other relevant areas to help partners start to process these experiences. During this processing, it's helpful if clinicians are aware of the partners' racial and cultural histories as a whole and how they can impact the couple. For example, if the partners are a South Asian Muslim couple, it is helpful that the clinician be aware of the racial, cultural, and religious tension between their cultures and how this may impact the couple, their families, and communities.

Ethical Nonmonogamy and Polyamory

An interracial/intercultural couple's relationship is diverse within itself; another intersectional experience of family structure involves ethical nonmonogamy and polyamory. Although interchanged in language, these relational and familial structures are different. Ethical nonmonogamy involves romantic and/or sexual relationships with an agreement between romantic partners to have additional partners (Brooks et al., 2022), is inclusive to romantic and sexual orientation, and is essentially an overall term for relationships that are not monogamous (Cardoso et al., 2021). Polyamory involves open relational practices, can be claimed as a relational identity, and refers to long-term, multiple romantic relationships with all members in the relationship involved simultaneously (Witherspoon & Theodore, 2021). At the essence of these relationships is consent, open communication, and rules that they abide by. Poly relationships make it abundantly clear that they are not deceptive partners, but rather all who are involved are on the same page.

What Is Ethical?

Ethics revolves around trust, fairness, and respect; these relationships thrive through transparency and shared ethical frameworks. Individuals in poly relationships may follow ethical principles such as equity of interpersonal feelings, freedoms of affection, dating, and love, and actions based on ideologies such as feminism or religiosity (Cardoso et al., 2021). These components also contribute to ethical dimensions of nonmonogomy and polyamory, which differentiates their relationships from infidelity or betrayal. For example, if their ethical framework is based on feminism, they may view their relationship as challenging patriarchal norms on sexuality, a renegotiation of gender roles, and advocacy of egalitarianism. A note here, both authors of this book identify as monogamous; thus, our positionalities are that of allies to nonmonogamous and poly relationships while maintaining a cultural humility stance, never fully knowing their experience.

There are various systems at play with nonmonogamy and poly relationships. At a micro level, individuals within their relationships are navigating their own sexual and romantic identities. For example, Bigner and Wetchler (2012) found that although gay men are in committed relationships, they may also be free to have multiple sexual partners. Conversely, Connolly (2012) highlighted lesbian women primarily focusing on emotional support and connection within monogamous relationships with ambiguity around open relationships. Lastly, although scarce in the literature, the LGBTQ community overall has overlooked nonmonogamy and poly communities. While sometimes placed under the umbrella of the LGBTQ identity, they may not identify as part of the LGBTQ community or identity.

Partners Creating and Navigating Their Own Relationship Rules

Historically, there has been a strong dominant narrative to monogamy and an even stronger adverse message toward infidelity. Many polyamorous couples need to work through negative messages of their attraction and relationship formation and provide levels of open education to their loved ones, describing not infidelity but rather an embracement of love. There is little literature regarding nonmonogamy and polyamory among interracial/intercultural/interfaith couples. Even in popular culture, messages celebrating monogamy over polyamory abound.

Rather, the structure of nonmonogamous and poly relationships are their own, and navigating the development of those relationships is a process individually and relationally. Microsystemically, partners may not be out to their family of origin due to fear or implicit messaging with lack of acceptance from them or religious communities (Rubinsky, 2018). On a mesosystemic level, those involved in the relationship will need to interact and engage following patterns from societal messages on relationships. While poly communities frequently face stigma in the larger community, they also tend to be heavily privileged and dominant in terms of Whiteness and power, excluding communities of color. In this way, polyamory may be considered a privileged space in the ability to have time and money to participate in open relationships, swinging, and related activities (Sheff & Smith, 2022).

It is our assumption that the relationship structures identified by Seshadri and Knudson-Martin (2013) and described below are relevant to how interracial and intercultural polyamorous dynamics are managed. However, we recognize that with multiple intersections involved between the interracial, intercultural, and interfaith partners and the therapist, a creative process with deliberate attention is needed, with explicit conversation and process regarding various dimensions of monogamy, open relationships, sexuality, attraction, and boundaries. While several movies and their sequels popularized and Hollywoodized BDSM and other types of sex, with hints of polyamory, it did highlight the negotiation between partners that sometimes may have to be formalized in a contract for protection. Such conversations may involve increased appreciation and love, but also increased stress and tension as these conversations may need to be continuously negotiated. More partners in the relationship suggest a need for more negotiation and advocacy between all relationship partners. Clinicians need to support equity processes around communication and negotiation so that all parties are heard and respected. As with all intercultural/interracial/interfaith relationships, it is advantageous for the clinician to have done their self of the therapist work in relationship to monogamy and nonmonogamy (see Chap. 2).

Welcoming Children and Parenting

Previous studies on interracial and intercultural families have primarily focused on racial classification and the problems of biracial children instead of parenting quality or techniques to help these couples that are already managing so much during this phase of life. The problem with racial classification is that it wasn't until the 2010 United States census that people were able to identify with more than one background. Fortunately, after 2010, practices are changing to slowly acknowledge multiracial backgrounds and other interracial-specific issues. What is most important is that biracial children have more stability when their parents can have constructive conversations around race, culture, and interreligious issues. Clinicians need to facilitate conversations around this by asking about how the parents talk about race, culture, and religion in front of the children, probing for age appropriateness and whether these conversations reach resolution, and if children have a framework for how they can talk about these issues. See Appendix 6.1 for more specific questions.

Roles and Division of Labor

For same-race couples, issues regarding gender roles and division of chores may be more hidden, especially during cohabitation, and may also change when children enter. However, once an interracial couple decides to have children, issues around tradition, meaning, cultural instruction, religious instruction, gender roles, and household labor take on added salience and must be overtly negotiated within the family. Because race, culture, and religion infiltrate instructions with gender, roles, etc., everything can take on a new meaning. For example, when taking the lens of race and culture, what is considered "equal" with household labor is nuanced by also racial and cultural histories.

Microsystem/Mesosystem/Exosystem

To understand how an interracial and intercultural family does parenting, we must explore their microsystem (experiences with parenting and stories around childrearing and how this affects the couple), mesosystem (how the couple's parents interact with them and around the children), exosystem (how the community responds to both the couple and the children), and macrosystem (societal messages to the couple and children). It is important for the White partner to acknowledge cultural influences on them and not just assume that only POC have culture. Interestingly, Lengyell (2020) also noted that the racial identity of each partner was re-shaped at the beginning of the interracial relationship, as well as with the appearance of a child, and during the school-age phase of the child. This can be especially challenging when the child is an infant when lack of sleep, stress, lack of or minimal support, and being first-time parents can be also part of the picture.

For school-aged children, how they are treated at school is based, in part, on their physical features (race), habits (culture), and traditions (faith), in addition to how other children interact with them (peer relations). History lessons, discussions around race relations, politics, and other educational topics such as migration/immigration, etc. are influenced by messages from the microsystem (parents), mesosystem (neighbors), exosystem/macosystem (school and the law).

With the recent political tension around education, for example, disagreements about whether or not to teach critical race theory or gender identity in schools/universities, interracial, intercultural, and interfaith parents and their extended families might have strong opinions about this and concerns for the impact on their children. For example, Hao, a 10-year-old, cisgender male, had his grandfather step into his school when the grandfather didn't agree with how Buddhist traditions were discussed in his grandchild's Christian school. Consideration of including extended families in treatment, as well as what is being discussed at school, is an important component of family structures. Clinicians need to be aware of how these factors can influence interracial, intercultural, and interfaith families/clients.

Though Seshadri and Knudson-Martin (2013) focused primarily on coupling (see Chap. 5), the various interracial and intercultural relationship structures they identified also apply to parenting. For example, they reported that the *integrated structure* organized their cultural differences in a way that melds both cultures together by celebrating each and differences are celebrated together. With parenting, for example, integrating traditions with baby showers or other traditions surrounding the celebration of the birth such as giving money to the family for the child. With *singularly assimilated*, one partner is more assimilated to the other's culture and isn't resentful about this; one culture takes a central stage. Extending the previous example, this could manifest as having a traditional baby shower based on one partner's traditions. In the *coexisting structure*, partners appear to retain their separate cultures, but they are rarely integrated. For these couples, differences are seen as positive and even attractive. These couples have two ways of doing many aspects of their lives (i.e., religion, parenting, spending styles, and childcare and/or household responsibilities) and appear to have an "agree to disagree mentality." For example, this would mean that the couple/family would have multiple baby showers representative of each background. Lastly, the *unresolved* structure describes couples not knowing what to do with cultural or racial differences and this being a source of conflict, where avoidance, tension, or outward resentment manifests. Essentially, it would be important for clinicians to help couples discover their relationship structure around their children and their relationship and move toward areas of adjustment based on the structure they desire vs what they currently have.

The Role of Parents

The impact of parents on their children's identity development is no surprise; parents are mirrors for their children as they communicate through their emotions, actions, body language, words, expectations, assumptions, approvals, validations, and rejections around race and culture explicitly and implicitly (Rockquemore & Henderson, 2010). Interracial and intercultural parents must deal with this from both sides of the extended family (Lengyell, 2020). When parents are supportive around racial and cultural identity development and socialization, especially in the home, they can have a positive impact on mental health and resilience in the face of discriminatory or prejudicial experiences (Corenblum & Armstrong, 2012). When specific family and racial/cultural combinations are not regularly discussed and ignored, as in the unresolved couple structure, the children struggle (Seshadri & Knudson-Martin, 2013). Killian (2013) also noted that it is important that partners who have privilege, regardless of the area of social location, make efforts to not show dismissiveness (either in humor or avoidance) toward the partner where there is a disadvantage. For example, if one is able-bodied and the other has a chronic illness, it's important for the able-bodied person to be affirming and embracing of the one with chronic illness and their management of it, especially in front of the children. Clinicians need to probe for processes around these issues and have direct conversations about them.

Microaggressions, insults that are related to race, gender, culture, class, etc. can also play a role in the dismissiveness of partners as well, even in humor (Williams, 2021). How microaggressions are interpreted is key; both when it's experienced and how it is responded to within the couple and the family. Accountability is important as well. Areas of negotiation between partners regarding childrearing include naming the children, discipline, education, food, chores, stances on medication/health, spending, and parenting style. Parenting can also bring up family-of-origin issues, especially related to culture and tradition. Furthermore, religion and spirituality also infuse these topics, as they give instructions for how people should live.

Blended Families/Remarriage

Older studies found that marriages between older Black and White couples were more likely to be remarriages from previous marriages to someone of the same race (Qian & Lichter, 2011). As with blended families, and depending on the age of the couple, therapists need to be aware of how to work with blended families/families of remarriage as well as how to treat interracial, intercultural, and interfaith dynamics, as they apply within the couple and family's intersections of identity (i.e., social locations). Clinicians need to extract how racial, cultural, and religious dynamics and expectations are influencing the family, depending on intercultural/interracial relationship structure, while including room for the blended and step-family dynamics; this is all in addition to helping the blended or step-family create a new family culture together (Papernow, 2018). Clinicians also need to explore how disadvantaged backgrounds influence the couple and how the couple can bridge the gaps between them. You can use Appendix 6.1 as a guide with step/blended families.

For example, in treatment with you, Lucy (cisgender, Hispanic female) would get mad at Matt (cisgender, White male) for being "too harsh" on her children when they didn't follow through with their chores. She expected him to let her discipline them (i.e., coexisting relationship structure), while he was trying to collaborate and be a part of the family or sometimes would expect her to discipline them the way he did his kids (i.e., integrated/singularly assimilated relationship structure). Through exploring her feelings, Lucy realized she was entangling cultural expectations, while also holding resentment regarding how he treated his own children from whom he was estranged. Through a lot of therapeutic work, they were both able to see that they were trying to operate with different relationship structures around parenting. If interfaith dynamics were also a part of this relationship, a good direction would be to explore how the couple incorporated spirituality/religion into their parenting and find a middle ground between their values and an agreed-upon relationship structure for handling their differences.

Fertility, Chronic Illness, Miscarriage

With more and more being discovered about fertility, children, and pregnancy, we need to briefly explore how fertility and miscarriage can affect interracial, intercultural, and interfaith couples. Qian and Lichter (2021) suggested implications for viability of fertility options based on race and the impact of chronic illness associated with race-based illnesses. It is important for the couple to have open conversations about their health history and the health trends that are race based (e.g., their race is prone to diabetes). Partners must acknowledge that as a parent, topics such as racial identity, racism, race relations, culture, and intersectionality must be discussed and are hard to avoid, especially when discussing pregnancy (Lengyell, 2020; Rockquemore & Henderson, 2010). If there is an unsuccessful pregnancy that results in an abortion or miscarriage, clinicians need to be ready to engage the couple in interventions and ways expressing grief and loss that are based on interracial, intercultural, and interfaith practices, and not limit this processing to only the female partner(s) (Samman et al., 2022). Clinicians need to address discourses around fertility, chronic illness, miscarriage, gender, grief, relationship expression, and communication. One way to do this could be through *remembering* which has origins of narrative storying and meaning exploration (Hedtke & Winslade, 2016). Olufowote et al. (2022) suggested using sociocultural assessments. Expanding on their research, we suggest the importance of exploring messages and discourses around grief and implications of blame on either relationship partner for whatever reason (e.g., illness).

All in all, a strength-based approach to learning about cultural differences and celebrations supports positive identity development for both the child and the family; mental health professionals need to guide parents to have these intentional conversations as it supports respect and value for each other's background (Lengyell, 2020; Seshadri & Knudson-Martin, 2013). This orientation provides more stability for children and promotes an environment where there are ongoing conversations where questions, negotiations, and comments can feel valid, respectful, and safe to have dialogue around.

Case Application

You worked with Eric and Lori, who came in not as most couples do. They were smiling and very loving with one another, which made you smile but also made you question "what is happening?" They started off telling you that they had been together for a long time, had four beautiful kids, a great sex life, and a strong love.

However, Lori (White, cisgender female, pansexual she/her) had come out as poly and wanted to open their marriage to involve an additional partner. Eric (Latinx, nonbinary, pansexual, they/them pronouns) knew the landscape of coming out, being part of sexually diverse communities, but was in uncharted waters on opening their marriage. Lori had already found someone she had emotionally connected with at a book club. Once these feelings developed, Lori came out to Eric and was completely transparent about who this person was, their love for them and their children, and wanting to work "it" all out. I couldn't help but admire and question how we would navigate our sessions. Eric seemed to accept Lori and was ready to work with her but they were tense, like something wasn't being shared.

After a while, it became clear that Eric had been pushing their feelings down deep to not hurt Lori; their mesosystem (Eric's family of origin) was directly and indirectly interwoven in their microsystem (marriage). Eric feared that once their family found out that Lori identified as poly and wanted to expand their relationship, they would never accept her or their marriage. His family was very traditional in their values in alignment with their culture. They believed that marriages were between two people; they attended church weekly and were quick to shame anyone who "steps out" on a marriage, which they viewed as a covenant beheld under God and the church. Although Eric's family was accepting of Lori's pansexuality and Eric's own identities, they felt there were boundaries they just couldn't further cross. They shared how grateful they were that a traditional Latinx family was accepting of his wife and their sexualities; how could they put more onto them? More for them to accept when they have done so much? However, Lori was asking the same questions—how could they not put more on them to unconditionally accept who Lori was and what their marriage would become?

This fear was immense. You witnessed Eric's shoulders tighten, their cheeks redden, their knee bouncing uncontrollably when they openly shared in session, and the stiffness to Eric's tone and hand motions, explaining that it would *never* be accepted. You were even intimated by this display. Funny enough, this didn't sound like the Eric you had come to know over a few sessions. The stiffness sounded like someone else. Through an experiential lens, you decided to deep dive into their family of origin rules, patterns, values, beliefs, and worldviews—particularly surrounding marriage.

First, you had to model a safe space for Eric, that the space you were creating and modeling for Lori was one that would be a nonjudgmental space for open dialogue. Unbeknownst to Lori, there was a strong culture of silence within Eric's family. One that felt "abundantly clear" as to what a marriage is and how it should represent the rest of the family. However, the rules of what marriage is need to be transformed in order for their marriage to expand and grow as they desired. All three of you worked on transforming rules into functional guidelines, paralleling the ethical framework of poly relationships. There was processing of awareness of expectations and silence to challenging traditional norms that may be harmful or restrictive. With Lori's support, Eric shifted "I can never share this" to "I can and need to share this." They did share eventually; their parents especially weren't happy and truthfully didn't understand. It created a shift in their system, a change that prompted fear and protection of their child from being hurt. However, after years of education, family sessions, communication coaching, and support, Eric, Lori, and their family continued the journey of acceptance and renegotiation of marriage rules.

Lessons from the Chapter

In this chapter, we discussed the act of marriage or making a long-term relational commitment and how marriage becomes a site of an evolving shared identity, especially when it comes to the integration of children. Rules and messaging from racial, cultural, or religious identity abound. Further, this becomes also nuanced when choosing to engage in nonmonogamy or poly relationships. Helping the couple own their own racial, cultural, sexuality, gender, and religious identity and how they want to intermix based on their relationship structure (integrated, singularly assimilated, or coexisting) will shape how they engage around children. Lastly, this will also shape pregnancy, fertility issues, chronic illness, and even miscarriage. Clinicians also need to be prepared to help families process grief based on interracial, intercultural, and interfaith interventions as appropriate.

Appendix 6.1: Marriage, Nonmonogamy, Children, Pregnancy with Your Interracial/Intercultural/Interfaith Clients

Note: Microsystem involves partners in the relationship, not just the couple regarding the referenced graphic

Microsystem (The Couple/Partners)- "We and the children"

Mesosytem- the couple and their friends and family ("We and what do they think of our family processes? (us)

Exosystem (the couple, their interactions with their own communities and culture. "We and how they support our children and us in the day to day?)

Macrosystem (the Couple and their interactions with society at large "we and how the world shows legitimacy of our relationship and our children") How do we deal with microaggressions?

Chronosystem (the couple and their interactions with time and pivotal events. "We and how this changes our family life")

The questions below provide a guided reflection across the ecological systems to inform your interventions with interracial and intercultural partners around marriage, non-monogamy, children, and pregnancy. Please complete this exercise after you have reflected and written down answers from Table 2.1. As you respond to the questions, please consider keywords from Table 2.1. For further exercise, imagine the graphic on this page, as a replacement of the top graphic in Appendix 2.1.

Microsystem—"We"

- What keywords do you notice about the couple's/partners' social location and identities in their discussions of marriage, nonmonogamy, children, pregnancy/fertility/miscarriage? What keywords or patterns do you see when you consider intersections of privilege or disadvantage?
- What keywords/meaning do you hear when the couple/partners discuss how they manage children, pregnancy/fertility/miscarriage? How do they negotiate normativity or nonnormativity when they integrate race, culture, sexuality, gender, or religion? Openness to nonmonogamy? How does this relate to their couple/family identity? How does this flow down to the children from their relationship structure?

Mesosystem—"Us"

- What stories or messages do you notice the couple/partners discussing when considering marriage, nonmonogamy, children, pregnancy/fertility/miscarriage, and their current or previous friends and family influence? How did/will you consider intersections of privilege or disadvantage?
- What traditions does the couple/partners have about culture, race, sexuality, gender, and religion from growing up? (Does this change based on the life stage of the family members?) How is this influenced by children, nonmonogamy, or any miscarriages? How much involvement does the couple/partners want to include other family members in their dynamics?

Exosystem—"Them"

- What messages do you notice the couple/partners discussing when considering marriage, non-monogamy, children, fertility, or miscarriage and their community influence? How did/will you consider intersections of privilege or disadvantage?
- What community messages (positive or negative) do the interracial, intercultural, and interfaith partners have about culture, race, sexuality, gender, and religion previously and currently in relationship to marriage, non-monogamy, fertility, pregnancy, or miscarriage (related to humor, specific events, acculturation, trauma, etc.) How do all of these stories of my interracial, intercultural, or interfaith clients influence their relationship with the communities that shape them?

Macrosystem—"World"

- What messages from government, advocacy, and social policy influence the interracial, intercultural, and interfaith partners around interracial marriage, non-monogamy, children, pregnancy, fertility, and miscarriage? How did/will you

consider intersections of privilege or disadvantage with the entities you have been associated with?
- How do historical or current laws and policies influence the stories of the interracial, intercultural, or interfaith clients around marriage, nonmonogamy, children, pregnancy, fertility, and miscarriage?

Chronosystem—"Life"

- What messages do you notice about the interracial, intercultural, and interfaith partners over the timeline of their relationship in how they address marriage, non-monogamy, children, pregnancy, fertility, miscarriage, and other macro messages about their relationship? With others? How did/will you consider intersections of privilege or disadvantage with the entities you have been associated with?
- How do they address bias, stereotypes, and other macro messages about their relationship? With others?

References

Amoateng-Boahen, G. (2015). The "culture of silence" contributes to perpetuating domestic violence: A case study of family life in the Brong Ahafo region of Ghana. Xlibris Corporation.

Bigner, J. J., & Wetchler, J. L. (2012). Gay male couple therapy: An attachment-based model. In *Handbook of LGBT-affirmative couple and family therapy* (pp. 45–62). Routledge. https://doi.org/10.4324/9780203123614

Brooks, T. R., Shaw, J., Reysen, S., & Henley, T. B. (2022). The vices and virtues of consensual non-monogamy: A relational dimension investigation. *Psychology & Sexuality, 13*(3), 595–609. https://doi.org/10.1080/19419899.2021.1897034

Cardoso, D., Pascoal, P. M., & Maiochi, F. H. (2021). Defining polyamory: A thematic analysis of lay people's definitions. *Archives of Sexual Behavior, 50*, 1239–1252. https://doi.org/10.1007/s10508-021-02002-y

Corenblum, B., & Armstrong, H. D. (2012). Racial-ethnic identity development in children in a racial-ethnic minority group. *Canadian Journal of Behavioural Science, 44*, 124–137. https://doi.org/10.1037/a0027154

Connolly, C. M. (2012). Lesbian Couple erapy. In Handbook of LGBT-Affirmative Couple and Family Therapy (pp. 63–76). Routledge.

Greif, G. L., & Saviet, M. (2020). In-law relationships among interracial couples: A preliminary view. *Journal of Human Behavior in the Social Environment, 30*(5), 605–620. https://doi.org/10.1080/10911359.2020.1732254

Hedtke, L., & Winslade, J. (2016). *The Crafting of Grief: Constructing Aesthetic Responses to Loss* (1st ed.). Routledge. https://doi.org/10.4324/9781315686806

Killian, K. D. (2001). Reconstituting racial histories and identities: The narratives of interracial couples. *Journal of Marital and Family Therapy, 27*, 27–42. https://doi.org/10.1111/j.1752-0606.2001.tb01137.x

Killian, K. D. (2013). *Interracial couples, intimacy, and therapy: Crossing racial borders.* Columbia University Press.

Lengyell, M. R. (2020). *Interracial couples and parenting: An exploration of interracial couples' experiences with parenting mixed-race children in the greater toronto area.* Retrieved from http://0-search.proquest.com.library.alliant.edu/dissertations-theses/interracial-couples-parenting-exploration/docview/2467465253/se-2

Olufowote, R. A. D., Samman, S. K., & Frick, H. (2022). Medical family therapy with diverse populations part II: Understanding & treating interracial & international couples with chronic illness using emotionally focused MedFT.

Papernow, P. L. (2018). Clinical guidelines for working with stepfamilies: What family, couple, individual, and child therapists need to know. *Family Process, 57*(1), 25–51. https://doi.org/10.1111/famp.12321

Patterson, K. (2018, January). The real truth about polyamory in the Black community. *Polyamory in the News By Alan M*. https://polyinthemedia.blogspot.com/2018/01/the-real-truth-about-polyamory-in-black.html#:~:text=%E2%80%9CI%20don%27t%20believe%20in,partners%20should%20all%20have%20autonomy

Qian, Z., & Lichter, D. T. (2011). Changing patterns of interracial marriage in a multiracial society. *Journal of Marriage and Family, 73*(5), 1065–1084. https://doi.org/10.1111/jomf.2011.73.issue-5

Qian, Z., & Lichter, D. T. (2021). Racial pairings and fertility: Do interracial couples have fewer children? *Journal of Marriage and the Family, 83*(4), 961–984. https://doi.org/10.1111/jomf.12758

Rockquemore, K. A., & Henderson, L. (2010). Interracial families in post-civil rights America. In *Families as they really are* (pp. 99–111). W. W. Norton.

Rubinsky, V. (2018). Revealing or Concealing Polyamory in the Family: Cultural Rules for Communicating Polyamory to Family Members. *Women & Language, 41*(1).

Samman, S. K., Frick, H. A., & Dansby Olufowote, R. A. (2022). Medical family therapy with diverse populations part I: Interracial couples navigating infertility, racialized pregnancy, and pregnancy loss. *International Journal of Systemic Therapy, 33*(4), 227–249. https://doi.org/10.1080/2692398X.2022.2125264

Seshadri, G., & Knudson-Martin, C. (2013). How couples manage interracial and intercultural differences: Implications for clinical practice. *Journal of Marital and Family Therapy, 39*(1), 43–58. https://doi.org/10.1111/j.1752-0606.2011.00262.x

Sheff, E., & Smith, H. A. (2022). Social class and polyamory. In *The handbook of consensual non-monogamy: Affirming mental health practice* (p. 315). Rowman & Littlefield Publishers.

Williams, M. T. (2021). Racial microaggressions: Critical questions, state of the science, and new directions. *Perspectives on Psychological Science: A Journal of the Association for Psychological Science, 16*(5), 880–885. https://doi.org/10.1177/17456916211039209

Witherspoon, R. G., & Theodore, P. S. (2021). Exploring minority stress and resilience in a polyamorous sample. *Archives of Sexual Behavior, 50*, 1367–1388. https://doi.org/10.1007/s10508-021-01995-w

Chapter 7
Navigating the Decades: Retirement and Expectations

I gladly took his last name. I've wanted it for a long time.

(Kantor, 2023)

A Seasoned Love

A quick search on the web yields minimal results for older individuals in intercultural relationships. In fact, the first three topics in our search read "Types of intercultural relationships," "Intercultural relationships: Entry, Adjustment, and Cultural definitions," and "Cross cultural relationships – dealing with differences." All of which long-term interracial, intercultural, and interfaith couples have navigated already for decades. However, when researching retirement, some interesting findings come through. There is resiliency in being together for decades and living in a society that has shifted acceptance, discrimination, and support throughout time.

A note here, both authors identify and have lived within a younger generation. We acknowledge the personal inability to fully capture older intercultural relationship experience; however, we stay curious, open, and advocates of older generations.

Chronosystem

In the modern day, interracial, intercultural, and interfaith relationships are being more accepted outwardly than previously, and those who may have not been able to be with their loved ones 60 or 70 years ago are now doing so. We see this in Jeanne Gustavson (White) and Steve Watts (African American). They are starting a new chapter; one of acceptance, reconnection, and freedom; they previously broke up due to Jeanne's mother's vehement disapproval of their interracial relationship when they were college sweethearts and reunited approximately 40 years later (Kantor, 2023). A clinician working with this couple would perhaps highlight interventions based on reconnection and reunification. Other seasoned interracial,

© American Family Therapy Academy (AFTA) 2024
G. Seshadri, D. Gutierrez, *Interracial, Intercultural, and Interfaith Couples and Families Across the Life Cycle*, AFTA SpringerBriefs in Family Therapy, https://doi.org/10.1007/978-3-031-58538-8_7

intercultural, and/or interfaith couples would be best served by exploring previous survival strategies around prejudice and discrimination.

Task: Legacy

Older individuals have gone through many experiences of life, through growth and wisdom and identity development. In this life stage, it's a process of finding joy and letting go of experiences younger generations can't imagine, celebrating history, acknowledging a loss of loved ones through miles, separation, and more prominently in older age–death. For individuals and couples who have gone through decades of life, there is often beauty in their experiences, grit in their fight, and love in their souls. Often the task at this life stage is one of processing and reflecting legacy (McGoldrick et al., 2013).

Macrosystem Influences: Existentialism, Religion, and Spirituality

Often during retirement and years after, individuals will take stock of their life as a part of their human experiences and make judgments and plans about how their life was meaningful or not, in connection with their hopes, dreams, and life goals. During this process of taking stock, meaning is attributed to legacy, which helps to ground the individual and feel like their life matters to future generations (Hunter & Rowles, 2005). They tell themselves a story of their life, which can increase meaning, connection, and communication with family and others and can also reflect their beliefs and values (Hunter & Rowles, 2005). Key events for interracial, intercultural, and interfaith couples can be moments of joy and distress; the negative part of this life stage may include facing feelings of loneliness, oppression, and feeling misunderstood, whereas the positive can be a celebration of difference and learning through relationship. This matters especially in cases of illness and existentialism, especially as the couple gets closer to what they perceive to be the end of their life. It is important to connect the couple to shared traditions, bridges of connection around religion, or even the opportunity to create traditions.

Task: Transcendence of Assimilation

When considering legacy, one reflects upon one's life and reviews ways of living. When it comes to interracial, intercultural, and interfaith relationships, partners may reflect upon how they "did or are doing" their relationship. Considerations and previous decisions around assimilation may be at play as a part of this review. In addition, seasoned older adults may feel more freedom to choose an interracial, intercultural, and/or interfaith relationship, as Jeanne did, and not have to worry about family of origin approval, especially with remarriage (Kantor, 2023; McGoldrick et al., 2013). Other reasons may include not having to worry about navigating race, culture, and religion with children, because their children have become adults and may not have to directly worry about this regarding influencing their mutual child's identity. Clinicians can probe for the current context with family approval and other considerations, including adult children and grandchildren.

What Are Considerations in Assimilation? Assimilation may be a potential experience and place of navigation for older interracial/intercultural relationships, depending on when they have moved to a new country. Sometimes older adults come to a new country to be taken care of by adult children. They may also be taking stock of this, due to changing life circumstances and opportunities, or when they are revisiting old life choices, and considering what they want their legacies to be, with the possibility of new meaning.

In general, if they are coming to a new country due to changing life circumstances, older adults may go through the traditional assimilation process. Assimilation is the process by which an individual or group adopts the customs, language, and behaviors of a dominant culture (Berry et al., 1989). To some extent, assimilation can be seen as a natural process that occurs as people adapt to new environments. It is not always linear and can be complex and ongoing. Additionally, not all individuals or groups follow the same trajectory, as assimilation can be influenced by factors such as social status, economic resources, and political power (Rumbaut, 2015; Sam & Berry, 2010). What constitutes assimilation has come under much debate and critique as it can portray diverse groups to eventually conform to the dominant as though it is inevitable or desirable.

Clinicians are advised to probe for adjustment and transition with assimilation and are encouraged to explore what this was like through the relationship or marriage for both interracial, intercultural, or interfaith partners. It may be helpful to create a timeline or even a cultural and/or religious/spiritual genogram. Old issues related to missed opportunities, loss, or regrets may need to be processed. It can also be a difficult process, especially for those who come from a marginalized or oppressed group. The pressure to assimilate can be intense, and it can be difficult to maintain a sense of identity while adapting to a new culture at a later age. In interracial relationships, assimilation can present challenges even though being born and raised in the same country. One partner may feel the need to assimilate into the culture of the other partner, leading to a loss of their own culture and traditions; this may be presented more prominently with intersectional identities within an intercultural relationship.

If they have previously assimilated, they may also be taking stock of this due to changing life circumstances and opportunities, or when they are revisiting old life choices and considering what they want their legacies to be, with the possibility of new meaning, they may go through a grief process related to missed opportunities, or reawaken old traumas from prejudice and discrimination that was experienced decades ago, and may be impacting the new relationship or transition. Through an ecological lens, assimilation has impacted and is integrated microsystemically and exosytemically.

Amalgamation (Marital Assimilation) and Ecological Systems Impact

As strong as seasoned love can be, this didn't come from minimal obstacles while the couple integrated their cultures and lives together. Strength and resiliency have been created due to years of an array of challenges and navigation of assimilation. Assimilation can be an important aspect of legitimacy for the interracial/intercultural/interfaith couple. Microsystemically, older couples may face social isolation, lack of support from family, and decreased community connection (Smith, 2012). Financially and economically, older children may not have the means to invite the older adults to live with them in their homes, or even have time to provide them with care. In interracial relationships, even as matriarch or patriarch of their families, they may also face rejection or disapproval from their family members. These experiences can be particularly painful on both sides (adult children and older adults), given the dedication and accommodations they may have given to their families throughout a lifetime.

Potential for Isolation: Mesosystem

Older adults may be isolated due to children moving out of homes, a shift to a home with accessibility, physical adversities, loss of mobility or community, and/or inability to continue living within their means, which can impact mental health (Sundström et al., 2020). Studies have found that older individuals experiencing isolation experience adverse mental health outcomes, such as depression (Gerst-Emerson & Jayawardhana, 2015). Differences in acceptance and their relationships can lead to misunderstandings, communication difficulties, and challenges to preconceived familial notions. It can be hard to continue to have the will to challenge these after so many years of life. Further, parent–child relationships will also carry prior history; this may influence communication and openness based on the old dynamics of the parent–child relationship.

Clinicians need to be aware of these parent–child dynamics and navigate carefully not only with the old issues but also recognize how the old issues may be augmenting the current lack of family approval and support around interracial, intercultural, or interfaith relationship or remarriage. There may be cultural, gender, and religious differences regarding expectations for intergenerational relationships, who provides care, and how is the younger generation expected to care for the older generation. In addition, are there implications based on cultural or religious beliefs around involvement or independence? There also may be cultural beliefs and practices around what happens to a parent's spouse when the other partner passes.

For example, Ramen (a cisgender, senior Singaporean male) is planning to get remarried to Clara (a cisgender, senior African American female). His children resist, in part due to disapproval of these types of relationships when his children were growing up. The children also have issues with the remarriage as they think it came too fast after their mother (cisgender, Singaporean female) passed away suddenly from a seizure, and were involved in their mother's care. They voice that they think Ramen is just trying to recapture his youth and didn't really love their mother. Ramen feels very connected to Clara, as his children moved away right after their mother's death, which he believes was to deal with the grief and loss of their mother. Themes of loneliness, connection, grief and loss, and chronic illness may be augmenting the racial and cultural issues.

Bridges of Connection: What to Do Within the Microsystem

It is helpful to consider how lack of usual means of connection and communication for some older adults can provide resiliencies in other ways. Interracial couples must get creative in how they shift from being "set in their ways" and navigate belonging or criticism within their own communities. These couples may get a unique chance to now rejoice in their diversity and intersectionality; a new chapter to renegotiate who they *were* to who they now *are*. Over time, there is often more of a prioritization of relationships and personal health over conflict and differences. This shift may contribute to greater emphasis on common experiences, shared values, and strong foundational relationships.

Further, although having the will to challenge may be much to muster, the chance to do so provides opportunities to role model embracement of change for younger generations. They can contribute to breaking down stereotypes, promote acceptance, and provide hope that change, love, and culture are to always be celebrated and can transcend cultural differences. Lastly, older adults in general have shown themselves to possess personal characteristics to contribute to openness to others and communities. These include exposure and familiarity, intergenerational relationships, and lifelong learning. This can be due to multiple factors, with the most prominent one being the amount of time that older adults have lived in a diverse community. With such an extended period of time spent in the community, there is exposure to experience with diversity and intersectionality either through friendship, romantic involvement, or demographic location over time.

The Exosystem: Challenges and Navigation of Culture

Exosystemically, older persons may face unique challenges in aging, including physical health problems and need of specialized care. Interracial, intercultural, and/or interfaith couples face an additional challenge of finding intersectional and culturally humble care. Care through cultural humility refers to healthcare that is responsive and respectful to cultural beliefs, values, practices, and traditions through understanding societal and contextual facts that influence cultural disparities and healthcare outcomes. With lack of support, adverse physical health experiences may come. For example, a study by Flores et al. (2012) found that lack of interpreters for non-English speakers, as well as no interpreters, led to significantly more errors and adverse clinical consequences.

Cultural communities may face obstacles finding clinicians and providers who would provide the care they need while understanding and accepting their identities. Further, finding care can be more of an obstacle for those couples that live in rural areas, who already face decreased access to mental and physical care (Henning-Smith et al., 2020). Interracial, intercultural, or interfaith partners need to learn how to be prepared to communicate on behalf of their partner or even with their partner's family around medical care, and may even have to participate financially, if able.

A final exosystemic factor revolves around media and connection. As noted, interracial, and intercultural relationships have become increasingly accepted. However, this doesn't come without strong prejudices and biases. While the media portrays a younger generation becoming more prominent in being discriminated against or fighting for equity, many older adults are facing the same experiences. However, due to the United States' cultures and prioritization of youth, their experiences may be sidelined. Further, they may have difficulties with cultural differences that, again, younger generations are learning and finding tools to communicate with; yet with adults who have grown and been shaped with core beliefs, discussing these differences may be much more difficult (Choi & DiNitto, 2013). Further, community connection for younger generations may come in the form of social media and events, yet connecting with older individuals or interracial couples is more of a struggle (Choi & DiNitto, 2013).

Retirement and Rediscovery: Mesosystem/Exosystem

Retirement can also be a place of connection for a couple. Often, this can occur simultaneously with an empty nest feeling when the last child moves away from home. The couple is often left to reconnect with each other without the influence of the children or their needs or activities. Often, what surfaces in retirement is a reconstruction of identity (McGoldrick et al., 2013). Role changes, awareness of partner's faults, impact of hobbies, and relationships with children are central themes. For the interracial, intercultural, and interfaith couples, while this is going on, a clinician would need to support ways of navigating conflict in these areas by finding previous solutions and reframes that enhance connection. It has also been suggested that retirement is most satisfying for couples when they both retire at similar times because they share the experience together, which seems to support togetherness and connection. In Europe, Comi et al. (2022) discovered that after retirement, men tended to keep colleagues as friends and females tended to reduce their friendship groups.

Suggested Interventions

Genograms can be helpful to explore topics such as acculturation, immigration, and migration stories, as well as experiences with dating, engagement, cohabitation, marriage, children, etc. (or the absence of these), which will tell stories across the generations. Use of a genogram can also highlight the importance of traditions, rituals, and symbols. Intersecting this with gender, socioeconomic status, sexuality, ability, and other social locations mentioned previously can add to the nuanced discussion for the couple on how they will navigate this life stage. In addition, clinicians can also help interracial, intercultural, and interfaith older adult partners create a positive legacy for themselves and help them to create goals that they want to connect themselves and each other to.

Clinicians may also want to help partners create a timeline of positive events from the past that they believe contributed to what they value and celebrate. Lastly, they may integrate scaffolding conversations to highlight what partners may already know about their stories to what could possibly be known. Asking questions around how to continue a positive legacy (e.g., language around commitment and joy), such as "What role will commitment and joy continue to play in your lives? How will you know that commitment and joy are loud and present in your heart and with one another?" Please see extended exercises in Appendix 7.1 for more.

Case Application

Joy, a 60-year-old Asian, Catholic, immigrant (now a full citizen), is now married to Hannah, a 70-year-old White woman who is Jewish and is struggling with cancer. They have been together for years; however, they were never able to legitimize their marriage or relationship due to the laws. They previously were married to heterosexual men of their own backgrounds. They came into therapy to seek support as Hannah was struggling with what direction to take her cancer treatment. Through generational genograms and family patterning, you discover that Hannah is going through an existential crisis and trying to make meaning of her life as she goes through her cancer treatment. Joy has always been pleasing and typically tries to fix things but feels helpless in not knowing how to take care of Hannah so that she becomes cancer free. She constantly searches the internet for treatments on how to cure Hannah's cancer and will engage in long debates with her on why she should consider the treatment based on the research that she finds.

Hannah initially indulged Joy; however, lately she is becoming angry and tired with the continual pushing that Joy does around the latest treatment measure that she finds. Both are estranged from their families, as when Joy came out, her family rejected her. You can relate to this as there have been estrangements in your family around culture in general and relate it to generational issues. Hannah's family is mostly deceased, but also had a strong dislike of Asian people, and when alive would engage in microaggressions toward Joy, which she would brush off. Through the process of therapy, you help the couple decide what meant the most to them was for Hannah to spend time at home with Joy together to make the most of the treatment; Joy felt that she could manage her anxiety better with Hannah being home and under her care. She (Joy) acknowledged that she had caregiver fatigue, but with Hannah being home, it felt more meaningful and spiritual to them that the shared time together, conversation, and a willingness to engage in legacy-based conversations helped them both to heal and grieve. Both were able to acknowledge and process the pain from their families, communities, and societal generational messages.

Lessons from the Chapter

In this chapter, we discussed how interracial, intercultural, and interreligious partners navigate the life stage of being older adults. What they must explore is how they can navigate legacy, connection, isolation, adult children, and existentialism. Helping partners create a positive legacy can help them distinguish the meaning they want for the future and from their past. Clinicians need to also be prepared to help families process grief based on interracial, intercultural, and interfaith interventions as applied to legacy, hope, and dreams. Extended exercises are included in Appendix 7.1. The central themes of this chapter are to honor differences as avenues of connection, provide support where there is loss, and find a middle ground in helping older adults assimilate as needed.

Appendix 7.1: Retirement and Older Couples

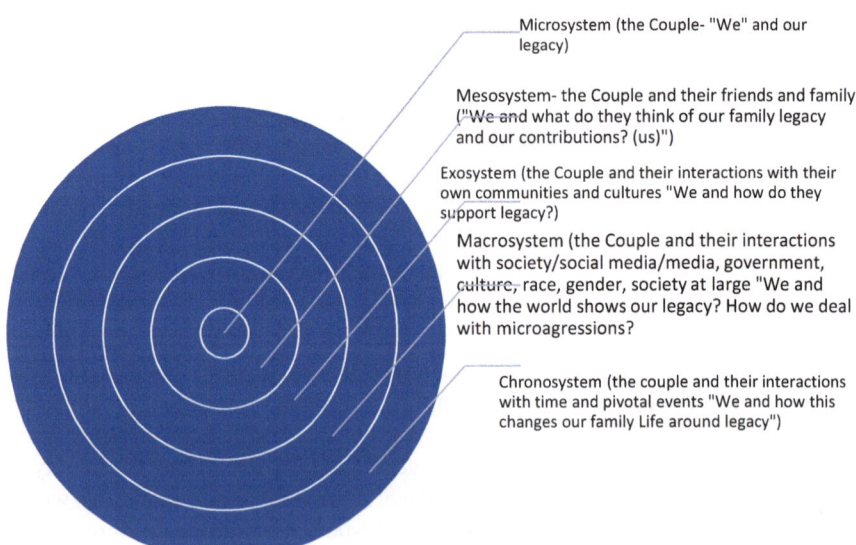

Microsystem (the Couple- "We" and our legacy)

Mesosystem- the Couple and their friends and family ("We and what do they think of our family legacy and our contributions? (us)")

Exosystem (the Couple and their interactions with their own communities and cultures "We and how do they support legacy?)

Macrosystem (the Couple and their interactions with society/social media/media, government, culture, race, gender, society at large "We and how the world shows our legacy? How do we deal with microaggressions?

Chronosystem (the couple and their interactions with time and pivotal events "We and how this changes our family Life around legacy")

The questions below provide a guided reflection across the ecological systems to inform your interventions with interracial and intercultural couples around retirement and aging. Please complete this exercise after you have reflected and written down answers from Table 2.1. As you respond to the questions, please consider keywords from Table 2.1. For further exercise, imagine the graphic on this page, as a replacement of the top graphic in Appendix 2.1.

Microsystem—"We"

- What keywords do you notice about the couple's social location and identities in their discussions of retirement, assimilation, connection, legacy, and existentialism? What keywords or patterns do you see when you consider intersections of privilege or disadvantage?
- What keywords/meaning do you hear when the couple discusses how they manage their adult children? What about assimilation, connection, legacy, and existentialism?

Mesosystem—"Us"

- What stories or messages do you notice the couple/family discussing when considering retirement, assimilation, connection, legacy, and existentialism and their current or previous friends and family influence? How did/will you consider intersections of privilege or disadvantage?
- What traditions does the couple have about culture, race, sexuality, gender, and religion from growing up? (Does this change based on the life stage of the family members? Grief? Assimilation?) How is this influenced by adult children, retirement, assimilation, connection, legacy, and existentialism? How much involvement does the couple/family want to include other family members in their dynamics? With rituals?

Exosystem—"Them"

- What messages do you notice the couple/family discussing when considering retirement, assimilation, connection, legacy, and existentialism and their communities' influence? How did/will you consider intersections of privilege or disadvantage?
- What community messages (positive or negative) do the interracial, intercultural, and interfaith partners have about culture, race, sexuality, gender, and religion, previously and currently in relationship to retirement, assimilation, connection, legacy, and existentialism (related to humor, specific events, acculturation, trauma, etc.)
- How do all of these stories of my interracial, intercultural, or interfaith clients influence their relationship with the communities that shape them?

Macrosystem—"World"

- What messages from government, advocacy, and social policy influence the interracial, intercultural, and interfaith partners around interracial retirement, assimilation, connection, legacy, and existentialism? How did you consider intersections of privilege or disadvantage with the entities you have been associated with?

- How do historical or current laws and policies influence the stories of the interracial, intercultural, or interfaith clients around retirement, assimilation, connection, legacy, and existentialism?

Chronosystem—"Life"

- What messages do you notice about the interracial, intercultural, and interfaith partners over the timeline of their relationship in how they address retirement, assimilation, connection, legacy, and existentialism? How do they address bias, stereotypes, and other macro messages about their relationship? With others?
- How did/will you consider intersections of privilege or disadvantage with the entities you have been associated with?

References

Berry, J. W., Kim, U., Power, S., Young, M., & Bujaki, M. (1989). Acculturation attitudes in plural societies. *Applied Psychology, 38*(2), 185–206. https://doi.org/10.1111/j.1464-0597.1989.tb01208.x

Choi, N. G., & DiNitto, D. M. (2013). The digital divide among low-income homebound older adults: Internet use patterns, eHealth literacy, and attitudes toward computer/internet use. *Journal of Medical Internet Research, 15*(5), e93. https://doi.org/10.2196/jmir.2526

Comi, S., Cottini, E., & Lucifora, C. (2022). The effect of retirement on social relationships. *German Economic Review, 23*(2), 275–299. https://doi.org/10.1515/ger-2020-0109

Flores, G., Abreu, M., Barone, C. P., Bachur, R., & Lin, H. (2012). Errors of medical interpretation and their potential clinical consequences: A comparison of professional versus ad hoc versus no interpreters. *Annals of Emergency Medicine, 60*(5), 545–553. https://doi.org/10.1016/j.annemergmed.2012.02.004

Gerst-Emerson, K., & Jayawardhana, J. (2015). Loneliness as a public health issue: The impact of loneliness on health care utilization among older adults. *American Journal of Public Health, 105*(5), 1013–1019. https://doi.org/10.2105/AJPH.2014.302427

Henning-Smith, C., Hernandez, A. M., & Hardeman, R. R. (2020). Rural-urban disparities in mental health outcomes among US adults with chronic health conditions. *Journal of Rural Health, 36*(2), 245–254. https://doi.org/10.1111/jrh.12416

Hunter, E. G., & Rowles, G. D. (2005). Leaving a legacy: Toward a typology. *Journal of Aging Studies, 19*(3), 327–347. https://doi.org/10.1016/j.jaging.2004.08.002

Kantor, W. (2023, February 3). A woman marries the love of her life 43 years after her mom pressured her to end interracial relationship. *People Magazine.* https://people.com/human-interest/woman-marries-man-43-years-after-pressure-to-end-interracial-relationship-real-life-love

McGoldrick, M., Preto, N. A. G., & Carter, B. A. (2013). *Expanded family life cycle: Individual, family, and social perspectives.* Pearson Higher Ed.

Rumbaut, Rubén G., Assimilation of Immigrants (2015). James D. Wright (editor-in-chief), International Encyclopedia of the Social & Behavioral Sciences, 2nd edition, Vol 2. Oxford: Elsevier, pp. 81–87, 2015, Available at SSRN: https://ssrn.com/abstract=2595896

Sam, D. L., & Berry, J. W. (2010). Acculturation: When individuals and groups of different cultural backgrounds meet. *Perspectives on Psychological Science, 5*(4), 472–481. https://doi.org/10.1177/1745691610373075

Smith, J. M. (2012). Toward a better understanding of loneliness in community-dwelling older adults. *The Journal of Psychology, 146*(3), 293–311. https://doi.org/10.1080/0022398 0.2011.602132

Sundström, A., Adolfsson, A. N., Nordin, M., & Adolfsson, R. (2020). Loneliness increases the risk of all-cause dementia and Alzheimer's disease. *The Journals of Gerontology. Series B, Psychological Sciences and Social Sciences, 75*(5), 919–926. https://doi.org/10.1093/geronb/gbz139

Chapter 8
Hot Button Topics: Can We Talk About Sex, Politics, and Religion?

It's important to have someone who is enthusiastically listening to and supporting you, and that you're not always having to be in an educational kind of mode.

(Schaefer, a Black man in an interracial marriage, New York Times, 2020)

The quote above applies to topics that all interracial/intercultural couples must navigate—sex, politics, and religion. With society already embroiled in marginalization against interracial and intercultural couples, decreasing perceived marginalization within their relationship may lead to greater integration of their relational and cultural identities (Yampolsky et al., 2021). However, these conversations may not be so easy. Interracial/intercultural partners may face clear racial and cultural and intergenerational differences, language barriers, and other processes that could create tension and distress. Kimberlé Crenshaw said it best, "We are a society that has been structured from top to bottom by race. You don't get beyond that by deciding not to talk about it anymore. It will always come back; it will always reassert itself over and over again" (Frontline, 2005, para. 52).

Sexuality

The term "sex" has various definitions to it. For this chapter, sex involves a combination of definitions including sexual expression, development, and intimacy. Hertlein et al. (2020) utilized a sexological systems model that discussed different sexual developments and experiences of relationships, a layer that interracial couples simultaneously navigate. With a foundation in ecological systems theory, sexological ecosystems examine the five systems through a sexuality lens: (a) microsystems involving biology of sexual stimulation and attraction and internalized messages of sex and gender from family of origin and peer groups; (b) mesosystems of individual sexualities blending together; (c) exosystems and societal messages of abstinence, sexual and body positivity, and culturally discriminatory health care systems; (d) macrosystems involving painful myths based in sex such as that men have higher sex drive than women; and (e) chronosystems such as history

© American Family Therapy Academy (AFTA) 2024
G. Seshadri, D. Gutierrez, *Interracial, Intercultural, and Interfaith Couples and Families Across the Life Cycle*, AFTA SpringerBriefs in Family Therapy, https://doi.org/10.1007/978-3-031-58538-8_8

of sexual assault, abuse, and traumatic experiences of sex and gender expression (Hertlein et al., 2020). Each system has been impacted by historical messages and events about sexuality.

Marginalization and Disadvantaged Voices

Embedded in history are myths and misconceptions of sexuality surrounding inter-racial/intercultural couples, such as perceived hypersexuality of POC or the idea that POC need to "move up" in status with White partners or same-sex interracial couples being sexually objectified (Naidoo & Lynch, 2020). Within Western culture, sex, and race are intertwined, where "accessibility to the bodies of Women of Color has a colonial legacy, rooted in perceptions that women of color are 'creatures of the flesh' who 'hide their pleasure' to fuel fantasies of invincible masculinity [Bhattacharyya, 1998, pp. 130–133]" (Buggs, 2017, p. 4). Within these historical premises, sex is deeply connected to power; for interracial and intercultural couples, power is an undertone that needs to be navigated.

For example, a vast amount of media and literature continue to portray interracial couples as White cisgender male and Black cisgender female, where there is a clear distinction of sociocultural power. Within interracial relationships with a White partner, Amy Steinbugler (2012) described gay, lesbian, and straight POC emotional labor needed to navigate discrimination, identity, and overall awareness/experience of oppression. She further emphasized this navigation being a silent process, one that partners may not be privy to, and particularly one that impacts sexuality and intimacy between partners. At their expense, POC partners may experience emotional exhaustion that can impact connection and sexual bonding (Steinbugler, 2012).

However, power involves much more than differences in race. It involves issues regarding culture, sexuality, gender, gender expression, ability, religion/spirituality, SES, and privilege. All of these identities and experiences are navigated within interracial/intercultural relationships; each with their own unique blueprints. What may be honored sexually in one experience may be limited in another. For example, Jose (cisgender male, Latino, heterosexual) and Yori (cisgender female, mixed race, pansexual) have been together for 1 year but are having trouble connecting sexually. Jose grew up in a home where his parents and grandparents did not speak of sexuality much. They emphasized marriage before having sex (presumed with a cisgender female), and as a teenager, he vowed chastity in his church group. However, any discussions on sexuality, sex or gender expression, or intimacy were not brought up or avoided. Jose mainly learned about sex through his peers and social media. Yori, on the other hand, had an upbringing very open to discussing sexual development and expression from a young age. Her parents were a resource and a safe space to come to for questions, as well as social support as she grew older. She had space and opportunity to explore her sexuality and came out as pansexual in high school. Both

Jose and Yori's sexual development and education, although different, were their experiences, and these need to be acknowledged by the clinician in order to help the couple figure out how they can honor both experiences between them without it being antagonistic because, on the surface, these appear to be opposite.

Bringing a societal context lens, a therapist working with this couple can help Jose and Yori acknowledge and process power imbalances in their relationship related to sexuality. Jose holds power as an identified heterosexual, cisgender man. He may unconsciously or consciously utilize his privilege to maneuver conversations on sex and sexuality, limiting or nuancing his history or how open he is on his experiences. However, Yori also holds power in the ability to put language and safety to sexuality discussions and have access to education throughout her lifetime. Sexuality and expression need both explicit and implicit conversation and co-navigation. Explicit conversations about sex, health, and boundary-making can serve as protective factors to individual and relational distress (Gómez et al., 2021). However, therapists need to be careful here as Yori, being part of intersecting, diverse identities, cannot be the only one providing space and education. Both Jose and Yori must acknowledge the power they hold and the privilege they can bring to their relationship regarding their sexuality as a couple. This can include asking about their sexual histories and questions revolving around how they explored their own sexual identities, intimacy, connection, and any cultural values that may be attributed to them.

Politics

The headline of a news article published in the Tennessee Tribune in 2022 headline read "Interracial Couples are Political, Interracial Marriages and Hate Crimes Are Increasing." The article interviewed well-known political researcher Justin Gest of George Mason University. Dr. Gest described how a relationship between the increase and acceptance of interracial/intercultural relationships paralleled an increase in racial and cultural prejudice in the United States. For example, a study by the California State University of San Bernadino Center for Hate and Extremism (2021) found that hate crimes, a form of external discrimination, against the AAPI community have increased by 169% since 2021. Politics have become binary and polarized; exosystemically, even without discussion, politics is already heavily embedded in their relationships. However, Dr. Gest went on to say, "When people intermarry it disarms the politics of polarization and division because those politics rely on very clean lines between groups" (The Tennessee Tribune, 2022, para 12). In the United States, clear lines have been embedded heavily in language including blue versus red, left versus right, liberal versus conservative. However, at the personal level, once interracial/intercultural couples have come together romantically, the lines become merged and they as a couple must navigate them. More specifically, the couple is actively engaged in their mesosystem.

Microsystem and Mesosystem

In review, the mesosystem involves interactions between microsystems; individual actions and behaviors are no longer isolated but intersect within their relationship. As a couple, their political ideologies are impacted by historical and present experiences and can contribute to their interactions, conversations, and presence with one another, not to mention the histories of previous generations and families of origin.

For example, Jones et al. (2011) highlighted variables that can impact the quality of interaction, including diet, stress, and social and cultural factors. For interracial/intercultural couples, variables can potentially be from historical and present factors. Further, in connection to racial discrimination, discrimination against sex and gender identity has also gone through civil rights movements for equity. Thus, relationships must negotiate factors of race, sexuality, and gender that have all come within political agendas. For example, as Yori identifies as mixed race and pansexual and Jose as Latino and heterosexual, both will never fully comprehend their experiences of discrimination or multiple microaggressions; however, this doesn't mean that they can't empathize or acknowledge each other's experiences. These experiences are merged into their communication of politics and policies that could impact their various identities. A therapist can guide couples in these conversations and stray away from polarizing ideologies, while acknowledging this underlying conflict as more than a superficial issue. For example, Jose couldn't fully understand having to choose between his parents around cultural issues and navigating this tension, or even Yori questioning initially why she liked those of multiple genders. On the other hand, Yori couldn't fully understand the pressures of being a heterosexual Latino male and assumed to be machismo, or other experiencing masculine pressures.

Minority Communities and Politics

In the United States, Black communities historically have been politically discriminated (i.e., racist politics) against through loss of human rights, equity, environmental inequality, and anti-crime policy. Other minority groups have also faced this form of discrimination with policies around immigration, abortion, gender, and sexuality. Civil rights movements such as the Black Panther Party were created and increased throughout time to combat political inequity. The fight continues to this day. For example, in the 2020 election, numbers of Black voters were turned away, waited in line for hours, had accessibility to only one polling center, and were exposed to state-controlled campaign media within certain electoral districts (Mutz, 2022). The Black Lives Matter movement has been not just for fair treatment under law enforcement but also a large political factor with politicians highly supporting or utilizing the movement as political gain (Boudreau et al., 2022). Tensions around these issues stem from trying to dismantle old ideas and replace them with more equitable policies.

How Do These Politics Affect Interracial/Intercultural/Interfaith Couples?

A study by Fall and Wittenberg (2022) interviewed seven participants in, or previously in, a Black-White coupling on their lived experiences as a couple regarding the United States social climate from 2020, particularly regarding political interactions with one another after the 2020 campaign. They found key themes regarding the impact of news, media, and politics. Participants described feelings of tension through voting, advocacy such as standing for the national anthem, and apprehension regarding police. For example, despite identifying as a White liberal person, their partner was upset that they didn't even take the time to vote. One other participant discussed their Black partner showing allegiance only to people of their own background when their national anthem was sung only causing tension between them. Politics are not only an issue with Black-White interracial couples; issues with other interracial, intercultural combinations can create stress as well, for example, with policies around immigration, regarding those that are undocumented, etc. It is important for a clinician to make room for both partner's voices; each of the partners needs to be empathized with, acknowledged, and heard from where they are coming from, as a starting point to then come to a mutual ground backed by their mutual values.

Many couples currently face unknown territory regarding how to navigate marked societal political divisions, with interactions involving feelings of anxiety, stress, and avoidance. Moreover, upticks in political division, including racial discrimination and microaggressions, have increased within the last few years. Partners may not want to rock the boat within their relationship, but knowing that there are clear differences in their political identity development and the impact of discriminatory experience is warranted. Some couples may avoid politics all together to sustain not only their individual mental health but also protect their relationship from outside political factors.

Recently, the political landscape has become more and more tense amongst conservatives and liberals. More and more people are specific about their dating preferences including political affiliation; for example, many have said that they will not even consider dating someone based on their political affiliation or even how they have voted on "hot button issues," such as women's issues, immigration, etc. (Easton & Holbein, 2021). Some online dating sites won't even list you if you are not willing to share your political affiliation. It has also become a divisive issue within families; cut-offs and estrangements may occur as family members feel misunderstood based on political choices. However, this issue, especially in the United States, has become unavoidable. Microsystemically, political differences and values need to be negotiated. Clinicians need to be aware of how lines were drawn in the beginning of the relationship politically, as this can influence trust and connection in the relationships, even if it's not being drawn amongst political party lines. Flexibility and shared values need to center the relationship and may even be the reason why they chose the interracial, intercultural, and interfaith partner from the beginning. It also may be necessary to gently and sensitively process why and how there can, or can't, be a middle ground between the partners on these "hot issues."

For example, Mandy (transgender female—she/her, Middle Eastern, liberal, agnostic) wanted to divorce Leslie (transgender Native American male—he/him, multiracial, conservative, Jehovah's Witness) over his unwillingness to get vaccinated during the COVID-19 pandemic. Through many sessions you were able to help the couple hear each other's reasonings and values around their positions; when drilling this down to process issues, however, in the end, it was Mandy who was closed off, as she had already decided she was ready to end the relationship due to not feeling heard for years around her intersectionality and wanted a relationship where she had a partner who shared her politics exactly. Leslie voiced feeling unheard as well around his beliefs and felt disrespected and frustrated with Mandy's lack of flexibility and angry resentment, leading him to give up. With these immovable stances, the couple mutually agreed to break up.

Religion

The Pew Forum on Religion and Public Life (2014) highlighted that 63% of people are in interfaith relationships. Often, religion has played a negative role in supporting interracial, intercultural, and interfaith relationships as we previously discussed (i.e. partners being unequally yoked, disrupting racial purity, and going against God). Further, racism and other policies have centered around preserving racial, cultural, and religious purity. Corinthians in the Bible/New Testament discusses that marital relationships should not be "unequally yoked" (Sossah, 2012). It has also been asserted that unequally yoked relationships are when there is a marriage between a believer and a nonbeliever in the teachings and principles of Jesus Christ; the premise is that they must be of the same religion for there to be equality within the relationship.

Avoidance

There are also other reasons why individuals avoid interfaith marriages; for many South Asians, this is due to concerns over intermarrying with religion and caste. As we have discussed in previous chapters, individuals continue to face societal and familial deterrents to interracial dating and marriage; adding religion to this mix also affects individual attitudes and to look at the choice to engage in these relationships as casual and not commitment worthy. Reiter and Gee (2008) studied interracial and intercultural couples and noted that religion was often not an area amenable to an open level of communication among dating couples.

From Hurdles to Connection

"Mixed" religion can create more hurdles for an interracial and intercultural couple and family to address. Familial pressure around these areas contributes to tension. However, clinicians can also make religion or interfaith dynamics a point of connection that complements personal values. Questions around mutual values and bridges of common ground are important to explore as well. For example, finding the value in both religions around being good people and connecting this to their attraction to one another.

Despite religiosity being a positive support mechanism for those that are believers in religion, spirituality, and God, a study found it was not enough of a buffer with a lack of support in relationship with depressive symptoms in interracial couples and families (Henderson & Brantley, 2019). However, also having the same religiosity, faith, or spiritual beliefs may be a form of connection regardless of racial or cultural differences. Clinicians must not be afraid to talk about these topics; it doesn't fall outside of the therapeutic relationship in terms of scope of practice (Reiter & Gee, 2008). Clinicians need to remember that they don't need to be in a place of quoting scripture etc., rather they are looking for ways to bridge values; for example, asking questions around how the two religions are similar and using that as a starting ground. Specific interventions are listed below along with additional exercises in Appendix 7.1.

The Mesosystem

In her research, Seshadri (2010) interviewed a couple and noted how this couple singularly assimilated their relationship structure around religion. Seshadri wrote:

> Samantha (White) assimilated to Juan's (Mexican) religion. Juan noted that her conversion was a part of his agenda, to "test and educate" her with religious questions because that is central to his family of origin's identity. Samantha sees this as positive: "Juan is the one who brought me back to the church, and introduced me to Seventh Day Adventist, the church, and really has taught me about it, because his family for many generations has been Seventh Day Adventist (Samantha, 254-258, #8)."

However, Juan stood up for Samantha when his mother demanded she be baptized in their church; he appreciated her assimilation but also decided to help set a boundary with his family. She appreciated this.

Families may fear that in intermarrying based on race, culture, and/or religion, their traditions, history, religion, allegiances to God and faith, and cultural totems or symbols will disappear. Transitions to sex/marriage/children may also reinforce the desire to be traditional within religion and other aspects of the relationship. Ideally, therapists create space to explore potential religious and spiritual assimilation. As seen with Samantha and Juan, Samantha noted the benefits of assimilation to "his agenda." Here therapists could explore and empower Samantha in assimilation and ensure Juan understands Samantha's journey into this religion, while honoring the history and value of religiosity for Juan. This would help promote equity of religious exploration in what otherwise might be a power imbalance in their relationship.

Exosystem and Macrosystem

Often, interracial, intercultural, and interfaith families get categorized as nontraditional and have been compared in terms of oppression to the experiences of LGBTQ+ individuals when they "come out"; side-by-side research has been encouraged (Perry & Whitehead, 2016). Since the LGBTQ+ populations have a negative history with conservatives and the church, these groups and individuals are likely to feel ostracized already. Perry and Whitehead (2016) suggested that both LGBTQ+ groups and interracial, intercultural, and interfaith couples and families may have similar experiences around religion. Similarly, through tradition, history, and scripture, it has been suggested that intermixing in race, culture, and religion goes against what are believed to be objective truths of religious communities; many communities have rejected LGBTQ+ or interracial individuals from frequenting their businesses in the local community based on objective personal beliefs based on religion.

It's hard to decouple religion from politics, sex, and relationships. Conversations between Yori and Jose need to center around similar values and common ground; since Jose hasn't had the opportunity to "come out" with intimacy, helping him talk about intimacy in ways he feels comfortable with is one way to start. Further, Yori may also come out to Jose in this relationship in ways that she feels comfortable. The clinician would help facilitate a nonjudgmental empathic attitude from both partners. As they both get into more of a pattern of give and take, this can help reduce the tension and perhaps the power struggle between them.

How Do We Navigate the Current Societal Discourse?

Patterns of interaction are largely based on family roles and rules and are regulated by boundaries serving to protect the autonomy of the family structure. Issues arise when restrictive family transactions and a family's structure have difficulty adjusting to changing circumstances. Thus, any change in the family structure may change the family worldview, and change in the family worldview will likely change the family structure. Clinicians can facilitate changes within family systems so that interracial, intercultural, and interfaith partners can promote macrosystemic changes within the organizations that they frequent. Challenging objective truths (i.e., rigid absolutes) is also another intervention. Such influences involve Western and international ideologies, assimilation and acculturation, restructuring of family structure (LGBTQ+ parenting duties, pressures, and roles), etc. Despite societal messaging pushing us in the United States to be polarized (i.e., Blue or Red), and like with Jose and Yuri, finding a common ground (i.e., the purple) is the best way to navigate the current discourses with hot button topics like religion, politics, and sex.

Case Application

Roy (age 33, Asian) and Randy (age 33, Black) are a cisgender gay couple who have been together for 13 years and just had a baby via surrogacy. They are both college educated and are seeking your services (i.e., couples therapy). Though they feel like they have solved their disagreements around familial conflict about the approval of their relationship, they are now considering how they would like to raise their child with racial and cultural differences. They have different ideas around how to explain their child's physical features that represent both of their races and whether the child should be religious, which has been causing significant conflict. When probing intergenerationally, you find that Randy's family history has deep roots in Christianity, and this was how his family through the generations survived enslavement, discrimination, and segregation. Roy's family spirituality was in Buddhism; he doesn't see the need for their child to be religious based on his frustrations with the church around their beliefs regarding the LGBTQ+ communities. Randy sees this as an afront to his family, and while he gets where Roy is coming from, still wants to raise their child with a Christian heritage.

Through intergenerational work regarding prejudice, grit, strife, advocacy, honoring elders, and discrimination and deconstruction of heteronormativity, the couple can recognize the values that they want to raise their child with. Further, through empathy and validation, the couple could explore and create advocacy for all communities involved (e.g., LGBTQ+; Buddhism; Christianity and family culture). While it was difficult initially to slowly unlock the coalitions that each had with their families and respective communities to find a common ground/shared values, the couple was finally able to hear the importance of each value, community, and influence of identity to the other. Lastly, they both voiced feeling comfortable with the shared history that they were going to be passing down their family line via their chosen families and traditions. They both agreed to have their child go with Randy to Randy's church (one that was accepting of sexual identity), still participate in advocacy with all the listed groups above, and agreed to share the importance of finding a surrogate who would represent Randy's racial background, as Roy was the donor for the surrogate. The values that they wanted to pass down to their child based on their common ground were acceptance, legacy and legitimacy of their relationship, and support.

Lessons from the Chapter

In this chapter, we discussed how interracial, intercultural, and interreligious partners navigate the sex, politics, and religion. As mentioned previously, while political issues can appear very binary, the goal is to bridge gaps between politics, religion, and other "hot button" issues, to find a flexible and common ground, often utilizing the qualities that may have initially attracted the interracial, intercultural, interfaith partners together. It is also helpful to recognize that while the impression and discourses (i.e., multiple realities) are that one must land amongopposites by picking a side (i.e., Black vs White, individualistic vs collectivistic, or monotheistic vs polytheistic), the reality is that all these issues are best viewed as a continuum. This enables relational connection and balance. Clinicians need to also be prepared to help families process slowly, especially when the common societal messaging is around polarization. Extended exercises are included in Appendix 8.1.

Appendix 8.1: Sex, Politics, Religion, and Other Hot Button Topics

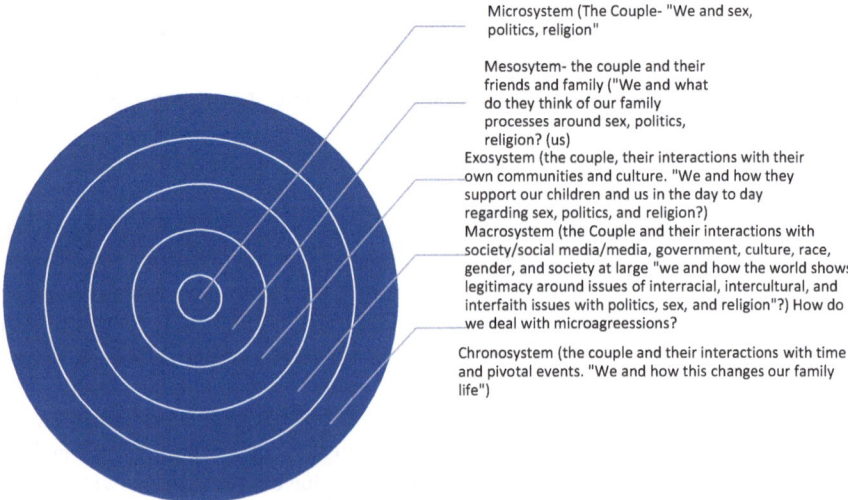

Microsystem (The Couple- "We and sex, politics, religion"

Mesosytem- the couple and their friends and family ("We and what do they think of our family processes around sex, politics, religion? (us)

Exosystem (the couple, their interactions with their own communities and culture. "We and how they support our children and us in the day to day regarding sex, politics, and religion?)

Macrosystem (the Couple and their interactions with society/social media/media, government, culture, race, gender, and society at large "we and how the world shows legitimacy around issues of interracial, intercultural, and interfaith issues with politics, sex, and religion"?) How do we deal with microagreessions?

Chronosystem (the couple and their interactions with time and pivotal events. "We and how this changes our family life")

The questions below provide a guided reflection across the ecological systems to inform your interventions with interracial and intercultural partners around hot button topics. Please complete this exercise after you have reflected and written down answers from Table 2.1. As you respond to the questions, please consider keywords from Table 2.1. For further exercise, imagine the graphic on this page, as a replacement of the top graphic in Appendix 2.1.

Microsystem—"We"

- What keywords do you notice about the couple's social location and identities in their discussions of sex, politics, religion, and other hot button topics?
- What keywords or patterns do you see when you consider intersections of privilege or disadvantage?
- What keywords/meaning do you hear when the couple discusses how they manage their shared values?

Mesosystem—"Us"

- What stories or messages do you notice the couple/family discussing when considering sex, politics, religion, and other hot button topics and their current or previous friends and family influence?
- How did/will you consider intersections of privilege or disadvantage?
- What traditions does the couple have about culture, race, sexuality, gender, and religion from growing up? (Does this change based on the life stage of the family members? Grief? Heteronormativity?) How is this influenced by sex, politics, religion, and other hot button topics?
- How much involvement does the couple/family want to include other family members in their dynamics?

Exosystem—"Them"

- What messages do you notice the couple/family discussing when considering sex, politics, religion, and other hot button topics and their community influence? How did/will you consider intersections of privilege or disadvantage?
- What community messages (positive or negative) do the interracial, intercultural, and interfaith partners have about culture, race, sexuality, gender, and religion previously and currently in relationship to sex, politics, religion, and other hot button topics (related to humor, specific events, acculturation, trauma, etc.)
- How do all of these stories of my interracial, intercultural, or interfaith clients influence their relationships and the communities that shape them?

Macrosystem—"World"

- What messages from government, advocacy, and social policy influence the interracial, intercultural, and interfaith partners around interracial sex, politics, religion, and other hot button topics? How did/will you consider intersections of privilege or disadvantage with the entities you have been associated with?
- How do historical or current laws and policies, influence the stories of the interracial, intercultural, or interfaith clients around sex, politics, religion, and other hot button topics?

Chronosystem—"Life"

- What messages do you notice about the interracial, intercultural, and interfaith partners over the timeline of their relationship in how they address sex, politics, religion, and other hot button topics?

- How do they address bias, stereotypes, and other macro messages about their relationship? With others?
- How did/will you consider intersections of privilege or disadvantage with the entities you have been associated with?

References

Boudreau, C., MacKenzie, S. A., & Simmons, D. J. (2022). Police violence and public opinion after George Floyd: How the Black Lives Matter movement and endorsements affect support for reforms. *Political Research Quarterly, 75*(2), 497–511. https://doi.org/10.1177/10659129221081007

Buggs, S. G. (2017). Does (mixed-) race matter? The role of race in interracial sex, dating, and marriage. *Sociology Compass, 11*(11), 1–13. https://doi.org/10.1111/soc4.12531

Center for the Study of Hate & Extremism (CSUSB). (2021). *Report to the nation: Anti-Asian prejudice & hate crime new 2020–21 first quarter comparison data.* California State University. https://www.csusb.edu/sites/default/files/Report

Easton, M. J., & Holbein, J. B. (2021). The democracy of dating: How political affiliations shape relationship formation. *Journal of Experimental Political Science, 8*(3), 260–272. https://doi.org/10.1017/XPS.2020.21

Fall, S. L., & Wittenberg, B. M. (2022). Experiences of White partners in Black–White romantic relationships in the United States: A qualitative study. *Family Relations, 71*(5), 2030–2046. https://doi.org/10.1111/fare.12778

Frontline Interview: Kimberle Williams Crenshaw, The OJ verdict. (2005). Retrieved January 25, 2024, from https://www.pbs.org/wgbh/pages/frontline/oj/interviews/crenshaw.html

Gómez, C. A., Kleinman, D. V., Pronk, N., Wrenn Gordon, G. L., Ochiai, E., Blakey, C., Johnson, A., & Brewer, K. H. (2021). Addressing Health Equity and Social Determinants of Health Through Healthy People 2030. *Journal of public health management and practice, 27*(Suppl 6), S249–S257. https://doi.org/10.1097/PHH.0000000000001297

Henderson, A. K., & Brantley, M. J. (2019). Parent's just don't understand: Parental support, religion and depressive symptoms among same-race and interracial relationships. *Religions, 10*(3), 162. https://doi.org/10.3390/rel10030162

Hertlein, K. M., Gambescia, N., & Weeks, G. R. (2020). *Systemic sex therapy.* Routledge.

Jones, K. E., Meneses da Silva, A. M., & Soloski, K. L. (2011). Sexological systems theory: An ecological model and assessment approach for sex therapy. *Sexual and Relationship Therapy, 26*(2), 127–144. https://doi.org/10.1080/14681994.2011.574688

Mutz, D. C. (2022). Effects of changes in perceived discrimination during BLM on the 2020 presidential election. *Science Advances, 8*(9), eabj9140. https://doi.org/10.1126/sciadv.abj9140

Naidoo, J. C., & Lynch, K. (2020). Global rainbow families: Examining visual depictions of same-sex couples in international picture books. *Bookbird: A Journal of International Children's Literature, 58*(4), 31–51.

Schaeffer, B. New York Times. (2020, July 2). *For interracial couples, advocacy is a love language.* https://www.nytimes.com/2020/07/02/fashion/weddings/for-interracial-couples-advocacy-is-a-love-language.html

Perry, S. L., & Whitehead, A. L. (2016). Religion and non-traditional families in the United States. *Sociology Compass, 10*(5), 391–403. https://doi.org/10.1111/soc4.12370

Pew Forum on Religion and Public Life. (2014, June 4–September 30). *Religious landscape study (RLS-II) topline* [Online forum]. Pew Research Center. https://www.pewresearch.org/wp-content/uploads/sites/7/2015/11/201.11.03_RLS_II_topline.pdf

Reiter, M. J., & Gee, C. B. (2008). Open communication and partner support in intercultural and interfaith romantic relationships: A relational maintenance approach. *Journal of Social and Personal Relationships, 25*(4), 539–559. https://doi.org/10.1177/0265407508090872

Seshadri, G. (2010). *How couples manage interracial and intercultural differences: What works?* (Publication No. 3415728) [Doctoral dissertation, Loma Linda University]. ProQuest Dissertations Publishing.

Sossah, L. (2012). Couples' experiences and perspectives on interracial marriage: A phenomenological study among adventists. *International Forum, 15*(2), 102–116.

Steinbugler, A. C. (2012). *Beyond loving: Intimate racework in lesbian, gay, and straight interracial relationships*. Oxford University Press.

Tennessee Tribune. (2022, August 11). *Interracial marriages are political: Interracial marriages and hate crimes are increasing*. https://tntribune.com/interracial-marriages-are-political/

Yampolsky, M. A., West, A. L., Zhou, B., Muise, A., & Lalonde, R. N. (2021). Divided together: How marginalization of intercultural relationships is associated with identity integration and relationship quality. *Social Psychological and Personality Science, 12*(6), 887–897. https://doi.org/10.1177/1948550620962653

Afterword: Concluding Thoughts

We intended this book to be a guide and helpful tool for therapists. With the use of ecological systems theory, intentionality with intersectionality, systems theory, and social constructionism, therapists can have important conversations with their interracial, intercultural, and interfaith clients to help them feel supported throughout their life transitions. With the added suggested exercises and visual representations of ways of integrating multiple theories with guided questions, our hope is that this offers additional tools to support interracial, intercultural, and interfaith partners.

With this systemic perspective and through time, the couple, family, community, and society can have strength-based experiences. While this book was intended for interracial, intercultural, and interfaith families who are heterosexual or identify with the LGBTQ+ populations, and with multiple areas of intersectionality of social locations, it can also be easily applied to transnational interracial, intercultural, and interfaith populations as well. Added stories, nuances, and conversations need to include immigration, visa processing, and migration stories, which ripple influence within all the systemic levels identified in Ecological Systems Theory.

We hope you found this work helpful in your clinical and research journeys; thank you for being a part of this journey.

© American Family Therapy Academy (AFTA) 2024
G. Seshadri, D. Gutierrez, *Interracial, Intercultural, and Interfaith Couples and Families Across the Life Cycle*, AFTA SpringerBriefs in Family Therapy, https://doi.org/10.1007/978-3-031-58538-8

Index

© American Family Therapy Academy (AFTA) 2024
G. Seshadri, D. Gutierrez, *Interracial, Intercultural, and Interfaith Couples
and Families Across the Life Cycle*, AFTA SpringerBriefs in Family Therapy,
https://doi.org/10.1007/978-3-031-58538-8